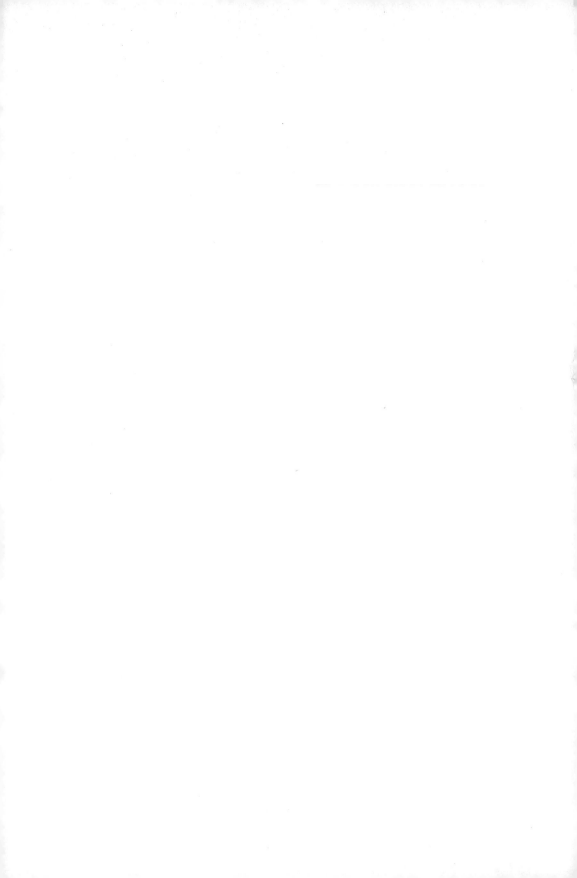

No More Pills.

No More Pills.

The Doctor-Approved, All-Natural Program for Reducing—Or Getting Off—Prescription Drugs

FROM THE EDITORS OF **Prevention**

with Martha H. Howard, MD, and Sara Altshul

RODALE.

© 2015 by Rodale Inc.

Prevention is a registered trademark of Rodale Inc.

Printed in the United States of America

Rodale Inc. makes every effort to use acid-free ⊗ recycled paper ♻.

Yoga workout photographs by Justin Steele;
other workout photographs by Mitch Mandel/Rodale Images

Book design by Carol Angstadt

Library of Congress Cataloging-in-Publication Data is on file with the publisher.

ISBN 978–1–62336–564–6 hardcover

2 4 6 8 10 9 7 5 3 1 hardcover

We inspire and enable people to improve their lives and the world around them.
For more of our products visit **prevention.com** or call 800-848-4735.

I dedicate this book to my husband, Gene; my children, Sarah, David, Andrew, Jason, and Adena; their partners, Thomas, Atyani, Anna, and Rachel; and my grandchildren, Michelle, Maxine, Oliver, Quinncy, Abe, and Asa; and to our youngest grandchild, who's due in April 2015. It is the love, support, and joy I feel in my life from my husband, children, and grandchildren, and my concern about their health, that inspired me to write this book. For the sake of my own family and all families, I hope to see a future that rejects the model of "disease management" (throwing pills at an illness) and makes true health care a reality.

—Martha Howard, MD

To my dad, Jack Altshul, a great newspaperman, who willed me his curiosity and his love for storytelling.

—Sara Altshul

Contents

Acknowledgments

I thank my coauthor, Sara Altshul, for all the fun of working together over the last 20 years, and for her great energy and great writing. I also thank Rodale Inc. for constantly providing the right information about all the "ingredients" of whole health. There just aren't enough words to say how much I appreciate all the resources Rodale provides for people who want to learn how to stay healthy.

I also thank Dr. Chris Costas, Belleruth Naparstek, Loretta LaRoche, Dr. Bernie Siegel, Dr. Francis X. Murphy, Dr. Leon Chen, Dr. Irina Tutunikov, Laura Lim, Gene Arbetter, Sarah and David Howard, all my patients, Loyola University Stritch School of Medicine (bless them for admitting me even though I was a woman in my late thirties and said openly on my application that I wanted to practice acupuncture!), Dr. Robert Carlson, and all my teachers at Loyola.

Introduction

In this book, Dr. Martha Howard and the editors of *Prevention* magazine bring to the table a new way of dealing with chronic illness. We hope you'll read this book cover-to-cover. We're confident that you'll discover strategies in these pages that will help you lower your dependence on medication, and by doing that, you'll be able to reclaim the health, energy, and sheer vitality that is your birthright. *No More Pills* is a research-based, doctor-tested program developed with Dr. Howard, a pioneering Chicago-based integrative physician who has dedicated her life to helping people recover from disease without drugs whenever possible. She will teach you how to heal using natural approaches including delectable food, mind-body techniques, gentle exercise and activities, herbs, supplements, and so much more. And you'll learn easy, drug-free, surprising, and time-tested strategies that will address the root of your problem. Think of this book as your antidote to 15-minute doctor appointments, and to physicians who are all too eager to prescribe the latest pill du jour.

Here are just a few highlights of the easy-to-use, drug-free, research-based recommendations you'll find within these pages.

Curcumin prevents diabetes progression. When 240 people with prediabetes were given either curcumin (turmeric) capsules or a placebo for 9 months in a 2012 study, none of the people who'd taken curcumin developed diabetes; 16.4 percent of the placebo group developed diabetes at the end of the study.[1]

Extra virgin olive oil slashes heart attack risk. In a 2013 study, people who used extra virgin olive oil as their main dietary fat slashed their risk of having a heart attack or stroke by 30 percent—and these were people at high risk for cardiovascular disease.[2]

Herbs ease arthritis pain. Taking a three-herb combination of devil's claw, turmeric, and bromelain (found in pineapple) for 15 days lowered the pain scores (with virtually no side effects) *by 30 percent* for people with osteoarthritis.[3] Black pepper and ginger have also proven helpful.

Blueberries lower blood pressure. Eating just one serving of blueberries a week makes you 10 percent less likely to develop high blood pressure than people who don't eat blueberries.[4]

Imagine Taking Fewer—Or No—Pills

The truth is that simple fixes like these aren't a topic of discussion at your doctor's office. And unfortunately, if you're like far too many Americans, you may already be taking a statin pill for your high cholesterol, one or more pills for your high blood pressure, or maybe a diabetes pill. In fact, millions of people with type 2 diabetes take insulin or another injected medication in addition to a pill. Is this really any way to live—by starting and ending the day taking handfuls of pills (or shots)?

Of course, we're not telling you to throw your pills out the window. That would be foolish—even life threatening. *No More Pills* offers a total lifestyle makeover that will help lower—or even avoid—the need for medications.

Why do we want you to get off the pills—or at the very least, be able to lower your dosage significantly? For one thing, most medications address symptoms and not the underlying illness itself. Having high cholesterol, high blood sugar, chronic pain, or high blood pressure, for example, is a symptom of underlying disease; it is not the disease itself. You can lower your high numbers and even your pain pretty successfully with medications—but you won't address the issues that caused your problem to begin with.

Furthermore, many medicines present side effects: Some cause fatigue, even depression; others, such as certain diabetes meds, have weight gain as their unintended—and insidious—side effect. Still others worsen inflammation, which is itself a chronic disease trigger. Pain meds can be addictive and pose the need for increasingly higher doses; other medications may interact with each other. Finally, there are the financial concerns to consider—depending on your insurance plan, your monthly pill bill may break your budget.

Once you decide to focus on reducing or losing your meds, you'll automatically start making healthy changes to improve your condition. Almost all of the chronic conditions we cover in this book, from arthritis to diabetes to IBS to sinusitis, can be improved with a diet of the right (and did we mention, delectable?) foods, an antistress plan, well-chosen supplements, and an action plan for increasing your physical activity.

Using stories from her case files, Dr. Howard will vividly illustrate how her patients have successfully beaten various disabling health problems, and she'll teach you how to enjoy the same kind of success from the comfort of your home.

Part I

Getting Off the Pills

Chapter 1

What's So Bad about Taking Pills?

The numbers are sobering: In 2012 (the last year for which we have statistics), 45,421 Americans died from side effects caused by prescription medications. By comparison, that same year, 16,000 people died in homicides, and 35,000 died in motor vehicle accidents.[1] Further, it's likely that the numbers are even higher than reported, because it's estimated that a mere 10 percent of all serious and fatal drug-related events are reported to the FDA. If you're wondering which drugs pose the greatest risks, it's blood-thinning medications that top the list for having serious—sometimes deadly—side effects.[2]

As Americans, we gravitate toward products that are "newer" and "better." This is especially true when it comes to drugs, because we—and our physicians—believe that the very latest scientific discoveries must certainly be improvements on yesterday's medicines.

But brand-new drugs are likely to be more expensive and, believe it or not, absolutely no more effective than those already on the market. Turns out, some 90 percent of all the new drugs approved by the FDA over the past 30 years are less or no more effective for patients than existing drugs, says Donald W. Light, PhD, network fellow at the Harvard University Edmond J. Safra Center for Ethics and professor at the Rowan University School of Osteopathic Medicine in Stratford, New Jersey.[3]

"The bar for 'safe' is equally low," writes Dr. Light in a Harvard University publication. "Every week, about 53,000 excess hospitalizations and about 2,400 excess deaths occur in the United States among people taking properly prescribed drugs to be healthier." According to Dr. Light, prescription drugs are the fourth leading cause of death in this country. And that's not even counting the some 80,000 "mild" side effects people experience each year without bothering to report them, such as aches, pains, digestive discomforts, sleepiness, and mild dizziness, says Dr. Light.[4] Even these minor reactions can mess with your productivity or functioning or, worse, can lead to falls and even to potentially fatal motor vehicle or other accidents.[5]

Sadly and scarily, studies can be biased, and important information is routinely misrepresented—what Dr. Light calls "institutional corruption." Pharmaceutical companies routinely hide, ignore, or misrepresent evidence about new drugs; distort the medical literature; and even lie about products to prescribing physicians, concludes Dr. Light and his coauthors in a 2013 article published in the *Journal of Law, Medicine & Ethics*.[6]

Those are some excellent reasons to have a serious talk with your doctor before agreeing to accept a prescription for some brand-new drug that's just come on the market. In fact, experienced, independent physicians recommend that you don't take a new FDA-approved drug until it has been out for 7 years, unless you absolutely must. That's the amount of time it takes to accumulate safety information, says Dr. Light.[7]

Is This Your Annual Physical?

Consider this information your wake-up call. I want you to create a knowledge-based partnership with your doctor—and to ask questions when she pulls out her prescription pad. Take this scenario, for example: You're 55 or 60 years old. You've just had your annual physical, and you're in the office again to get the results of your lab tests. Your doctor informs you that you're 15 or so pounds heavier than you were last year (and you thought the dry cleaner shrunk your favorite size 12 slacks). But there's worse news. All your numbers are edging into the red zone—your blood sugar is high, and so are your blood pressure and cholesterol.

Here's what's most likely to happen: Your doctor will tell you to lose some weight, get some more exercise, and come back in 6 months for retesting. Some doctors, depending on just how high your numbers are, may diagnose you as having metabolic syndrome or prediabetes and may even start you on medications right away—as many as three different pills—to get your levels back to normal. Making sure your levels are back to normal sounds like a healthy move, but is it really?

Turns out, when it comes to prediabetes, the costs and potential side effects of diagnosing people with and medicating them for this "condition" may actually not be worth it, says a 2014 study by researchers from University College London and the Mayo Clinic.

"Prediabetes is an artificial category with virtually zero clinical relevance," says lead author John S. Yudkin, MD, emeritus professor of medicine at University College London. "There is no proven benefit of giving diabetes treatment drugs to people in this category before they develop diabetes, particularly since many of them would not go on to develop diabetes anyway," he continues.[8]

I agree completely with the authors of the study. It's yet another example of our broken diagnostic system, which generates this trifecta: a "defining" lab test, a disease label, and a for-profit pharmaceutical solution—instead of any attempt to deal with all of the real aspects of this constellation of health problems.

It's absolutely true that many people in the United Kingdom and the United States—not to mention other countries around the world—are walking time bombs for diabetes. And it's equally true that giving a drug to people physicians label as "prediabetic" on the basis of a single lab test is no solution to their problem. In fact, I believe there's a huge potential for harm. Taking a pill encourages people to continue in their same old habits of poor diet and too little exercise. They think continuing these unhealthy habits is "safe" because the pills will protect them from harm. Their blood glucose may look good on paper, but if they don't make real changes in their diet and activity habits, they, like most people, will likely progress right on to full-blown diabetes.

What does work for people whose lab tests put them in the prediabetes range? A community-oriented prevention program might actually help prevent diabetes. The combination of learning how to eat more healthfully (which, by the way, doesn't mean missing out on delicious food), learning how to incorporate more activity into your day, and getting some social support has been proven as effective as medication in stopping prediabetes in its tracks. Taking that pill doesn't give you a chance to turn things around, according to the results of the study.

What Should Happen?

In a perfect world, during that second visit to review your lab results, your doctor would send you home with a journal to record your eating, sleeping, and exercising habits along with your stress levels and would urge you to come back in a month to review all your entries. If you were in my office, I'd also be testing you to see whether you have delayed-type food allergies to wheat, dairy, and other foods. Once the results were in, I'd recommend a diet that's better suited to your needs, an activity plan, and some stress-reduction exercises. I would check on your social and emotional support systems and would make sure you have the appropriate support.

I'd encourage you to stick with this plan—maybe even referring you to a nutritionist for some eating education and to a trainer to help you create an exercise regime you'll commit to. (I might even refer you to a Diabetes Prevention Program, like the one many YMCAs offer for free, which incorporates all of those elements.)

My method of treating chronic problems like diabetes starts with "treating the root." This means that I'd investigate all of the potential factors that contribute to your problem. I'd help you resolve them so that your body (and your mind and your spirit) comes back into balance. We'd start with the basics.

- Food (see "What Are You Eating?")
- Water
- Environment
- Exercise
- Sleep
- Stress reduction
- Social and spiritual support

What Are You Eating?

When a patient comes into my office, I ask lots of questions—probably more questions than most people are used to getting from their doctors. The answers help me figure out what steps we need to take. One area I question very closely is the patient's diet, because in my experience, that's where most people need to begin in order to improve their health and start feeling better. Below are the kinds of questions I'd ask. Since you're not in my office right now, I suggest that you get out a piece of paper and answer the following questions.

Q. What's the quality and quantity of food you're eating every day?

Q. Check the choices that mirror your eating habits.

___Grabbing a toaster pastry on the way out the door

___Hitting a fast-food drive-thru and eating in your car

___Snatching a greasy deli muffin with your creamy, sugary latte

___Wolfing down a sandwich in 10 minutes flat at your desk

Q. Once home and exhausted, do you put away a bag (or two) of microwave popcorn in front of the television?

Q. Are you eating too many cold, sweet, or processed foods?

Q. Do you react to common food proteins, such as gluten (wheat and other gluten grains) and dairy (casein)? Symptoms can include diarrhea, abdominal discomfort, nasal congestion, and headaches, for example.

If you're still not feeling better after we've addressed these key issues, then I'd likely recommend some herbs or other dietary supplements and potentially some acupuncture.

In My Office

If you're on the track toward developing diabetes, these are some of the steps I might take.

First, once I understand what you're eating, I'll help you optimize your diet to make sure you're getting plenty of foods and snacks that have been proven helpful for lowering blood sugar and improving other diabetes markers. For example, I'd make sure you're eating at least a couple of servings of tasty pistachio nuts or almonds every day. Here's why: Two 2014 studies revealed that these nuts can lower both blood sugar and insulin resistance.[9]

I would also give you a good curcumin supplement, made from a compound in the yellow curry spice turmeric. When people diagnosed as prediabetic were given only 250 milligrams of curcumin a day for 9 months, *none* of them progressed to full-blown diabetes.[10] In the control group of people who took a placebo, 16.4 percent of them progressed to diabetes. This study of 240 people was conducted in Thailand and published in *Diabetes Care*, the journal of the American Diabetes Association.

Also, I would give you two herbal supplements known to lower glucose, berberine and bitter melon. I recommend 500 milligrams berberine two to three times a day and 500 milligrams bitter melon once a day. I'd then have you back regularly every month to check on your progress and figure out what is and isn't working for you so I can edit your program. We'd keep track of your blood sugar for 9 months. If your test results show you edging back toward health, then yay for you—keep up the good work! No pills needed.

But sadly, I'm afraid that what happens in my office happens in only a minority of doctors' offices across the country.

Just Ask: Why?

I want you—and your doctor—to ask one question, which is the missing link, I believe, in our health-care system. Why? Why did your blood test results show such unhealthy numbers? And why are you experiencing vague problems—such as insomnia, sugar cravings, irritability, painful joints, fatigue, trouble concentrating, digestive difficulties—problems you can't really label but that make your life less fun to live?

The answer isn't that you're lazy. The answer is that the modern American lifestyle you're probably leading simply isn't conducive to your health. I won't tell you that there's some giant conspiracy among fast- and processed-food companies (including giant beverage makers), mega-entertainment corporations, corporate agribusinesses, chemical manufacturers, and, yes, even the pharmaceutical industry to keep Americans like you fat, happy, and hooked. That would be crazy talk. But I can tell you that given the avalanche of advertising and other messages we Americans get about products and activities that don't support our health, it's difficult for many of us to change our approach to living the healthy life we were meant to live.

Chronic Disease Isn't Normal

These days, having a health condition such as high blood pressure, heart disease, arthritis, high cholesterol, or diabetes has become a sad rite of passage for all too many American adults. These and other chronic problems are driven largely by our couch potato culture, processed-food diet, and sedentary jobs. As a result, we are more overweight than ever before—which makes us prime targets for many largely preventable lifestyle diseases.

Unfortunately, with a medical system that lacks a focus on prevention, it's all too easy for time-stressed doctors to prescribe pills that you're expected to take for the rest of your life.

If you ask me, our American medical system is almost completely focused on disease management, rather than on health care or prevention. And I'm afraid that most doctors confuse "prevention" with premedication or early detection.

Here's what I mean: Giving statins to otherwise healthy people as "prevention" for heart disease has not been proven effective. In other words, we have no scientific proof that taking a statin in the absence of having heart disease will actually prevent a heart attack. And what's worse, we've recently learned that doing so may put people at greater risk for diabetes or for muscle pain and damage.[11]

I believe that our current level of "pill pushing" is completely out of hand and connected with a broken diagnostic system that fails to seek the causes of disease. Instead, it assigns a disease label to a set of symptoms and then prescribes pills, procedures, or both. It's almost like a high-tech version of the old barber-surgeons who used knives, bleeding, leeches, cautery, arsenic, and laudanum (slash, burn, and poison) instead of gentler (and more effective) healing techniques, such as herbal medicine, to name just one.

The Shape We're In

One of the driving forces that led us to creating this book is the fact that so many Americans are suffering from one or—all too often—*several* different chronic diseases. It's no secret that we don't get enough exercise and have less than healthy diets; both are huge factors when it comes to promoting chronic illness. And the most recent statistics paint a stark picture of where we're going off the rails, health-wise. The numbers are positively alarming.

- As of 2012, one in four American adults has two or more chronic conditions; 50 percent have one or more.[12]

- Seven of the top 10 causes of death in 2010 were caused by chronic disease—of these, heart disease and cancer accounted for nearly half of all deaths.

- One out of three American adults is obese.

- Of people ages 65 or older, 45.3 percent have two or more chronic health problems.

- Of people ages 45 to 64, 21 percent have two or more chronic health problems—and the numbers are growing.

- Death related to pain medications tripled between 2000 and 2010.[13]

- Fifty percent of Americans take prescription drugs.[14]

- Use of antidepressants increased to more than 10 percent of the population.[15]

- Americans spent $263 billion on prescription drugs in 2011.[16]

- In 2011, 52 percent of American adults didn't get enough aerobic exercise or physical activity.

- Thirty-eight percent of Americans say they eat fruit less than once a day, and 23 percent eat vegetables less than once a day.

- One in five Americans is still smoking cigarettes, which accounts for 480,000 deaths each year. And 38 million adults say they "binge drink" on a weekly basis, having an average of eight drinks per binge. Yet most binge drinkers aren't alcohol dependent.[17]

Breaking the Drug Cycle

When your doctor says you need to take a medication for your chronic illness, chances are you're going to listen. That's because at least 70 percent of us have confidence in our doctors' advice, say the results of a Gallup poll taken a few years ago.[18]

But it might be a wise move to ask your doctor what else you might be able to do first—such as tweaking your lifestyle habits—before you begin taking a drug. Make no mistake, the purpose of this book isn't to tell you that prescription drugs are always bad or harmful. Instead, what I'm hoping you'll learn is which chronic conditions are somewhat within your control and what you can do to lessen your dependence on prescription drugs.

The following numbers really should stagger all of us. According to a 2013 report (based on data collected between 2007 and 2010) from the Centers for Disease Control and Prevention (CDC):

- 48.5 percent of us used at least one prescription drug in the past 30 days.

- 21.7 percent of us used three or more prescription drugs in the past 30 days.

- 10.6 percent of us used five or more prescription drugs in the past 30 days.

- 79.3 percent of all visits to a hospital ER were linked to reactions caused by drug therapy.[19]

It's interesting to take a look at the top 10 drugs—and the conditions doctors treat with them—that were prescribed between April 2013 and March 2014. Some of the drugs on this list (see page 14) may seem surprising to you.

Even "Benign" Drugs Pose Problems

I n my 30-plus years of practice, I've seen countless people who've been medicated for conditions that could be better treated with a cleaner, more natural diet of mostly organic, nonprocessed foods; more physical activity; relaxing mind/body practices; and appropriate supplements and herbs—all of which I'll discuss in later chapters of this book.

Of these conditions, four top the list for being some of the most frequently diagnosed. Sadly, as I've mentioned, when most doctors make a diagnosis of one of these "big four" conditions, they may only mention those essential healthy lifestyle recommendations to their patients in passing, if at all.

Unfortunately, the first-line drugs prescribed for these conditions—drugs we usually think of as benign—can actually cause insidious side effects. Some of these side effects have been apparent for some time; others we're only recently discovering.

Here's a brief look at four of the major chronic problems we face most frequently and the frontline drugs that are commonly prescribed for them when the disease is first diagnosed.

Condition: High Cholesterol

Causes: Poor diet, excessive weight, heredity, age, gender.

Drug problems: Statin drugs prescribed to lower cholesterol can cause muscle pain and, more rarely but seriously, a condition called rhabdomyolysis, which is a breakdown of muscle tissue. Statins have also recently been linked to causing diabetes.[20, 21]

Condition: Diabetes

Causes: Excessive weight, poor diet, inactivity, heredity.

Drug problems: Metformin is just one of the many drugs prescribed for diabetes. It's currently thought by many to be a benign starter drug for almost everyone newly diagnosed with type 2 diabetes. Recently, however, we're learning that metformin might cause issues with memory loss. Other commonly mentioned side effects of metformin can include taste problems, headaches, nausea, vomiting, diarrhea, cramps, bloating, and lowering vitamin B_{12} to inadequate levels.[22]

Condition: High Blood Pressure

Causes: Aging, excessive weight, poor diet (especially one high in salt), inactivity, certain medical problems such as chronic kidney disease, heavy drinking, smoking, and side effects of some medications.

Drug problems: Hydrochlorothiazide raises blood glucose and may also cause dizziness, nausea, vomiting, and diarrhea, among other problems.[23]

Condition: GERD (Gastroesophageal Reflux Disease)

Causes: We used to call this condition heartburn or acid indigestion, but now it's become an official disease. GERD is one of my pet peeve "label diagnoses." Most often, GERD is gastritis or esophagitis caused by a delayed-type allergy to food proteins. I have had literally hundreds of patients over the years who'd been, in my opinion, misdiagnosed with GERD. Happily, I've been able to take them off proton pump inhibitors (PPIs) when they made the dietary changes I recommended. But that's a rare treatment plan these days, when most doctors overlook functional causes and instead prescribe these expensive drugs, often for years on end. Now, we're beginning to discover that PPIs have long-term side effects.[24]

Drug problems: Recently, experts have raised concerns over these drugs, which were once considered quite safe. For example, they appear to affect vitamin and mineral absorption and may lead to the development of iron-deficiency anemia and other vitamin and mineral deficiencies, including B_{12}, calcium, and magnesium. What's more, emerging evidence suggests that people who are in the early stages of PPI therapy may also be at higher risk for pneumonia.[25]

DRUG	CONDITION	NUMBER OF PRESCRIPTIONS
1. Synthroid	Thyroid problems	23,025,870
2. Crestor	High cholesterol	22,868,588
3. Nexium	Heartburn, GERD	19,327,244
4. Ventolin HFA	Asthma, bronchitis	17,503,208
5. Advair Diskus	COPD	15,545,755
6. Cymbalta	Depression, anxiety	14,487,742
7. Diovan	High blood pressure	12,017,281
8. Vyvanse	ADHD	9,914,366
9. Lantus SoloStar	Diabetes	9,858,068
10. Lyrica	Pain conditions	9,578,165[26]

A Surprising Fact about America's Most Prescribed Drug

I was a little surprised to discover that Synthroid, the synthetic thyroid hormone, is America's most prescribed medication. But its popularity points to a problem I've long been warning my patients about: the fluoridation of our water.

I believe that one reason for the massive number of people suffering from hypothyroidism—a condition in which people lack sufficient thyroid hormone (and the primary reason behind all those Synthroid prescriptions)—is that we routinely add fluoride to our public drinking water. And although the CDC listed water fluoridation as one of the "10 great public health achievements of the 20th century," facts are emerging to suggest fluoridation simply isn't the great health benefit we once thought it was.[27]

Let's step back and review the history: At the turn of the 20th century, an American dentist from Colorado became aware of patients whose teeth were mysteriously stained. He also noticed that people who lived in areas where stained teeth were common also had remarkably lower rates of dental decay.[28]

A statistical comparison of 4,000 children ensued. It turned out that people living in the areas where stained teeth were most common did, in fact, have many fewer cavities. Enter Alcoa, the Aluminum Company of America. Because the staining had occurred in Bauxite, Arkansas, where Alcoa mined much of their aluminum, it was feared there might be a link between the staining and the leeching of aluminum into the drinking water. However, testing revealed that the one common factor all the stained teeth sites shared was higher than normal levels of fluoride in the water. The conclusion? High levels of fluoride in drinking water lead to lower levels of dental decay.[29]

In the mid-1940s, cities around the country began adding fluoride to public water; several studies followed that confirmed that fluoridation reduced cavities significantly.[30]

Cut to the present day. In 2006, the National Research Council (NRC) issued a report. It stated that the Environmental Protection Agency's safe drinking water standard of 4 parts per million (ppm) of fluoride puts people at—wait for it—an increased risk of tooth damage. And that's not all— the report also noted that it puts people at greater risk for bone damage, too.

And what about the thyroid disease connection? Well, according to that same NRC report, there's evidence to show that fluoridation affects thyroid function. The report goes on to say that fluoride exposure in humans is linked to elevated levels of thyroid-stimulating hormone. And when TSH is elevated, it means the thyroid gland isn't producing enough thyroid hormone. Synthroid to the rescue!

Most (97 percent) Western European countries do not add fluoride to their water systems, and yet tooth decay has dropped as sharply there as it has here in the United States. This suggests to me that fluoride has nothing to do with our vastly improved dental health. And in Japan, which bans fluoride, officials have stated that "fluoride may cause health problems."[31]

Bottom line? Our overzealous water fluoridation program has had the unintended consequence of exposing millions of Americans to thyroid problems.[32, 33, 34]

Dealing with Fluoride

I recommend to my patients that they remove fluoride from their water and stop using dental products that contain fluoride. The best way to do so is to purchase a good water filter and use it as directed. I like the APEC Water Countertop Reverse Osmosis Water Filter, available from Amazon for $229. It's very effective at removing fluoride and other contaminants and, as a bonus, needs no installation. A less expensive option is the Seychelle water pitcher, at $48 from Amazon. It removes about 85 percent of the fluoride.

A Look at America's #2 Drug: Statins

Yes, prescription drugs can save your life. But what's the cost—to your health and to your wallet? Let's take a look at statins, the second most commonly prescribed class of drugs in America.

Once your doctor diagnoses you with high cholesterol, she may suggest you begin taking a statin drug. Cholesterol, a waxy, fatty substance, is a key recipe ingredient for building cell membranes and for making hormones, including estrogen and testosterone. About 80 percent of the cholesterol your body needs to function is made in your liver; the rest comes from the meat, poultry, eggs, fish, and dairy products you eat (plant foods contain zero cholesterol). When your diet includes too many foods that are cholesterol-rich, excess cholesterol—remember, it's waxy and fatty—deposits itself along the interior walls of your arteries, narrowing and weakening them. That leads to high blood pressure and atherosclerosis (your granny likely called it hardening of the arteries), which substantially raise your heart attack and stroke risk. For more about cholesterol, see Cardiovascular Disease on page 138.[35]

Now, a new study confirms what I've long suspected. Turns out, one unintended consequence of prescribing statins to lower high cholesterol is that they seem to offer people a false sense of security that subtly encourages them to eat too many calories and fatty foods, say UCLA Health Sciences researchers. The researchers compared people who took statin drugs during 2009 to 2010 with people who took the drugs 10 years earlier. They discovered that people taking statins a decade ago consumed fewer calories and less fat than people who didn't take the drugs, and they also learned that statin-takers today have a higher body mass index compared with statin-takers 10 years ago.[36]

"We believe this is the first major study to show that people on statins eat more calories and fat than people on those medications did a decade earlier," said the study's primary investigator, Takehiro Sugiyama, MD, who at the time of the study was a visiting scholar at the David Geffen School of Medicine at UCLA. The 2014 study, "Gluttony in the Time of Statins," was published in the *JAMA Internal Medicine* journal.[37] "We believe that when physicians prescribe statins, the goal is to decrease patients' cardiovascular risks that cannot be achieved without medications—not to empower them to put butter on steaks," said Dr. Sugiyama.

This statement is one I wholeheartedly agree with, and it is at the core of this book: Yes, there will be some people for whom drugs such as statins can be lifesaving. But the first step toward wellness will always be through eating healthfully, getting active, and managing stress. Yes, some people who are dedicated to living well will still have to take medication—in some cases, maybe more than one pill. But drugs should rarely be our frontline treatment. What you'll learn in these pages is how to use diet and other good-for-you approaches that will inevitably reduce your reliance on drugs.

Statin Side Effects

As I've noted, it's true that statin drugs can lower cholesterol and improve the health of many people who are prone to dangerously high cholesterol levels. But in addition to the unintended consequence of increasing your consumption of fatty foods, statins also pose side effects—though it's also true that only a relatively small percentage of people will experience them.

Recently, the FDA updated its advice about statin risks. "The value of statins in preventing heart disease has been clearly established," says Amy G. Egan, MD, deputy director for safety in the FDA's division of metabolism and endocrinology products. "Their benefit is indisputable, but they need to be taken with care and knowledge of their side effects."[38] These include:

Memory loss. The FDA has been studying reports of memory loss, confusion, and forgetfulness from statin use. The FDA notes that these reports span all statin drugs and occur, albeit rarely, across all age groups. According to Dr. Egan, these experiences can include feelings of "fuzzy" or unfocused thinking, and they have occurred in people who've taken the drugs for 1 day or for years. Symptoms weren't serious and apparently disappear after a few weeks of discontinuing the medication.

Type 2 diabetes/increased blood sugar. Your doctor will most likely monitor your blood sugar levels after you've started taking statins. That's because, according to some reports, there's a small risk that higher blood sugar levels and even the development of type 2 diabetes could occur with statin use, says the FDA.

Muscle pain. According to the FDA, some drugs interact with statins to include the risk of myopathy, which is a muscle injury that causes unexplained muscle weakness or pain. This occurs because these drugs are metabolized through the same pathways that statins follow, which increases the amount of statins in the blood—and the risk of muscle injury. You may experience muscle pain as an ache, soreness, or weakness in your muscles, ranging anywhere from an annoying discomfort to a severe pain that gets in the way of your daily activities, such as going up or down stairs. Know that some medications interact with lovastatin and can increase the risk of muscle damage, says advice from the FDA.

Muscle damage. An extremely rare, but extremely serious statin side effect (usually limited to people who take high doses of statins or those who take statins in combination with other drugs) is rhabdomyolysis. Symptoms include liver damage, muscle weakness, stiffness, and soreness; it can also cause decreased urine output or dark-colored urine. Notify your doctor at once if you experience any of these symptoms.

Liver damage. Before the FDA warning, it was standard procedure for doctors to monitor your liver enzymes via blood tests before (and/or during) statin therapy. The new FDA guidelines say that doing so isn't necessary after all, because monitoring hasn't been effective for predicting—or preventing—the rare cases of serious liver injury linked to using statins.

Digestive discomfort. Rarely, people experience nausea, gas, diarrhea, or constipation while taking statins—but usually, people who get these upsets have other digestive issues.

Rashes/flushing. If you also take niacin or a statin drug that contains niacin, such as Simcor, you could flush or have a rash shortly after taking your meds.[39]

The Dangers of
Prescription Pain Medications

There's an American drug abuse epidemic raging today, and it's affecting three groups of people you'd never associate with addiction: senior citizens, stressed-out moms, and even children (it's also the running subject of the popular cable TV show *Nurse Jackie*). The problem? Prescription painkillers. Deaths from painkiller overdoses have never been higher, says the CDC. In fact, nearly three out of four prescription drug overdoses are caused by these drugs, which are also known as opioids.

Sales of these potentially lethal drugs have risen more than 300 percent since 1999, and in 2008 they caused 14,800 deaths—more than cocaine and heroin combined. More than 475,000 ER visits were attributed to opioid misuse and abuse. If a new virus began infecting and killing Americans at these rates, you can bet that researchers would be jumping all over themselves to find a vaccine (and big pharma would be drooling to get its hands on the patent).[40, 41]

Even you can become an addict. Here's an example of how easy—and how doctor-sanctioned—it is: Say you've developed sudden knee pain that persists until it really slows you down. You check in with your doctor, get an

Is This Your Sleeping Pill?

It's unfortunate but true that millions upon millions of us regularly have trouble getting a good night's sleep. If you're among them, turn to Insomnia on page 212, where I'll outline a pill-free program to help you get all the restful slumber you need. In the meantime, here's an emerging public health alert about the popular prescription sleeping pill zolpidem (Ambien). The troubling fact is that hospital ER visits from zolpidem overdoses *nearly doubled* to more than 42,000 in 2010; 68 percent of these visits were by women. In fact, adverse reactions to this drug were so common that in 2013, the FDA lowered the recommended dose for women by 50 percent.[42]

"When zolpidem is combined with other substances, the sedative effects of the drug can be dangerously enhanced," according to the 2013 report from the Substance Abuse and Mental Health Services Administration (SAMHSA). People with the largest proportion of zolpidem-related ER visits were between 45 and 54 years of age, noted the SAMHSA report.[43]

The bottom line is, I don't want to see you taking sleeping pills like zolpidem; it's my goal to help you discover natural ways to drift off to sleep. But if you are taking the drug, stay safe: Follow your doctor's directions exactly, and never combine zolpidem with opioid drugs, other sedatives or sleeping pills, or alcohol.

What Else Is in That Pill?

When you read the label of a drug or a supplement, the ingredients you focus on are the active ones—the actual medicines. But I want you to also be concerned about those ingredients labeled "inactive" (called *excipients*), especially if you have food sensitivities. Because guess what? Inactive doesn't translate to "won't cause problems."

In fact, people can and do have problems with these supposedly inactive excipients. I've had patients with corn, soybean, and milk allergies experience allergic reactions to pharmaceuticals and even to over-the-counter medications that contained ingredients to which they were allergic. Problem is, these patients had no idea the pills contained substances they'd normally strictly avoid.

Lactose, which is a milk sugar, has reportedly caused serious allergic reactions when people with severe milk allergies used asthma inhalers that contained lactose fillers. Soy protein isolate is another excipient that could cause people with soy allergies to react severely.[44] Several years ago, the *New England Journal of Medicine* reported the cases of two women, ages 58 and 81, who experienced dangerously low blood pressure and difficulty breathing after taking a generic version (omeprazole) of the popular prescription antacid Prilosec. It turned out that the drug contained soybean oil; both women were allergic.[45]

The remedy for this is to read supplement labels with a magnifying glass, if necessary. And if you're taking a prescribed drug, talk to the pharmacist to make sure it doesn't contain substances to which you might be sensitive.

x-ray, and are told you have "a little arthritis." You're sent home with a prescription for a strong nonsteroidal anti-inflammatory drug.

A week or two later you're still hurting, so you see an orthopedic specialist. She looks at the x-ray, sees the arthritis, and injects some cortisone into your knee. When it wears off and the pain returns, back to her you go. This time, she schedules you for an MRI. It turns out that you have a common knee injury known as a torn meniscus, which is a rip in the C-shaped cartilage that surrounds your knee.

The doctor recommends arthroscopic surgery, which she says is a simple, uncomplicated procedure using tiny instruments; the surgery takes an hour or so and will barely leave a scar. You'll be up and around in a couple of days, she assures you.

But you're not. In fact, after 2 days of severe pain (despite your prescribed opioid pain medications, such as Percocet or Vicodin), you're in worse pain than you were before the surgery. Your doctor may recommend physical therapy, but for the next month or even longer, while you're dealing with pain that's as bad as ever, she'll continue to renew your opioid prescription. And now you're discovering that while the pills don't actually make the pain go away, they do make you care a little less about feeling it. So you're taking the pills as directed, and while you're not actually "high," you do feel a pleasant little buzz that you'd like to keep on feeling. And there you have it: the birth of an addiction.

You may find it easy to put down those pills; you may not. Eventually, if you're like most of us, you'll simply be too embarrassed to ask the doctor to refill that Rx yet again. But if you've really become hooked, you might turn to illicit means to score more of those little white pills.

Here's what should happen instead: First, some meniscus injuries can heal on their own, given the right kinds of activities. So that's the route I'd take initially. Ask your doctor for a referral to a good physical therapist. Then, I'd make sure you were eating a diet high in anti-inflammatory foods, and I'd see to it that you were taking an appropriate dose of curcumin, along with some Chinese herbal formulas, and getting acupuncture and tui na (a Chinese massage technique). I'd also recommend some water exercise, such as an aqua aerobics class, which many Ys and fitness centers offer.

Nutrition: Where Wellness Begins

The reason why doctors are so quick to prescribe drugs rather than help you transition to a healthier way of life comes down to one thing: their training or, should I say, their lack of training in what I believe is the single most important aspect of wellness, nutrition. The paltry amount of time American medical school students spend training in nutrition—when our obesity and diabetes epidemics are virtually out of control—would be laughable if it wasn't so pathetic.

Nathaniel P. Morris, a second-year Harvard Medical School student, published a June 2014 editorial in *JAMA Internal Medicine* that described the education he'd received in nutrition at that point in his med school career. Compared with the 60 classroom hours of cardiology instruction he and fellow students received during their second year in med school, Morris says his nutrition training "spanned just three afternoons, for a total of 9 hours of classroom instruction." Morris learned that those 9 hours would be the only exposure they'd get to nutrition education during their 4 years of med school. No exams, no interactions with patients. Their only obesity lecture was just 45 minutes long.[46] Shocking? You bet. Remember, we're talking about a leading medical school in a country where one out of three people is obese.

Harvard is by no means the only med school giving short shrift to this essential public health topic. In his editorial, Morris cites a 2010 study of 109 medical schools, which revealed that the state of nutrition education has barely changed, if not deteriorated, in the 25 years since a National Academy of Sciences report on this topic. As of the 2010 report, of all 127 accredited medical schools, only 25 percent required a dedicated nutrition course, and the average amount of nutrition education was down to 19.6 hours.[47]

"The amount of nutrition education that medical students receive continues to be inadequate," says the author of that study, Steven H. Zeisel, MD, PhD, the Kenan distinguished professor of nutrition and director of the Nutrition Research Institute at the University of North Carolina, Gillings School of Global Public Health in Chapel Hill.[48]

Now, compare med schools' 19.6 hours of nutritional education to what naturopathic students receive at Bastyr University in Kenmore, Washington. Naturopaths are doctors whose medical education is as long and as demanding as that of conventional MDs. But instead of studying illness management, naturopaths study "wellness management." To that end, the Bastyr curriculum requires *126.5 hours of nutritional education.*

Even if your current doctor isn't as well versed in nutrition as you might wish, not to worry. In the chapters that follow, I'll give you the kind of nutritional know-how you need to set yourself on the path to healing. Following the suggestions in Chapter 3, plus the specific suggestions in Part II, based on conditions you may be battling, will help. If you need more support, seek out a nutritionally savvy health care professional who can give you the additional help you need.

Finally, if you're worried that the No More Pills Plan is going to separate you from the delectable foods you love, let me put your mind at ease, because nothing could be further from the truth. You'll enjoy meats, seafood, eggs, and a rainbow of vegetables and fruits. And don't forget the desserts! How about marinated fruit, crustless apple pie, ice cream, pudding, and, yes, even cookies. Instead of white flour, you'll discover how delectable nut flours are for all your baking needs. Cocoa powder is allowed, eggs are allowed, and as far as meals and snacks are concerned, that's flexible. It's whatever suits you best.

For Your Consideration: Traditional Chinese Medicine/ Acupuncture

If you're committed to taking a more natural approach to your health, you may want to consider enlisting the aid of a healer who is trained in techniques that don't rely on pills to cure disease. My personal favorite is traditional Chinese medicine (TCM).

In use for some 3,000 years, traditional Chinese medicine isn't just a combination of exotic healing techniques; it's a completely different healing philosophy, one that takes a 360-degree turn from conventional Western medicine. TCM is near and dear to my heart—I've trained in traditional acupuncture, laser acupuncture, and Chinese herbal medicine; and before I received my medical degree at Loyola University Stritch School of Medicine, I got a master's degree at Harvard University in Chinese language and literature. I also served as a board member for 3 years of the American Association of Acupuncture and Oriental Medicine. So I'm extremely comfortable sharing my favorite medical philosophy with you.

We "treat the root" in TCM. Remember, that means we look at all of the factors contributing to your health problem and work toward resolving them until you've achieved a state of balance that's right for you.

(continued on page 26)

The No More Pills Plan Could Prevent or Improve Alzheimer's Disease

As I was writing this book, I came across an exciting study entitled "Reversal of Cognitive Decline: A Novel Therapeutic Approach," published by Dale E. Bredesen, MD, director of the Alzheimer's disease program at UCLA's David Geffen School of Medicine in 2014 in the journal *Aging*.[49]

Dr. Bredesen and his team created a personalized, therapeutic approach—much like the No More Pills Plan—that combined diet, exercise, and specific supplements. The therapy was designed to improve the mental deterioration associated with Alzheimer's disease and other dementia-related conditions.

Each of the 10 participants had aspects of the program tailored specifically to them, but some elements were common to all.

1. They eliminated all simple carbohydrates from their diets.

2. They increased consumption of fruits, vegetables, and nonfarmed fish and followed a strict meal pattern with specifically timed interludes of fasting.

3. Exercise was a key component, and participants also decreased stress through practices like yoga and meditation.

4. Participants took many daily supplements, including fish oil, vitamin D_3, coenzyme Q10, melatonin, and others.

5. Where appropriate, female participants resumed previously discontinued hormone replacement therapy.

Here's the amazing outcome: At the time of this writing, 10 people had been studied. Prior to beginning the program, six of them had had to quit working or were struggling at their jobs; after completing the program, all were able to return to work or continue working—with improved performance.

The great news is that these people have continued to show improvements as far out as 2½ years after their initial treatment. Trust me, no pill exists that can even come close to results like this. It's really miraculous.

"What this program says is that we are all contributing to our own Alzheimer's disease by the diet we choose to eat, by the way we sleep, by the stress we have in our lives, by our microbiome, and of course by our genetics," said Dr. Bredesen. He went on to say that we can alter our cognitive decline by changing those factors in our lives.

Virtually every aspect of the UCLA program matches what we do in the No More Pills Plan—except that we also determine whether you're having delayed-type food reactions to your diet. We therefore enable you to put an end to food-related body-wide inflammation that contributes to the degenerative aging process.

Let's take a look at just one of the study's successful case histories. A 67-year-old woman came to the research team after experiencing 2 years of progressive memory loss. She held a demanding job that involved preparing analytical reports and traveling widely, but she was having trouble analyzing data and writing the reports and was afraid she'd have to quit her job. She couldn't remember her reading material, forgetting what she'd read by the time she reached the end of a page. She even had to write down four-digit numbers to remember them. And she had trouble navigating on familiar roads, often getting lost. She also mixed up the names of her pets and forgot where the light switches were in the home she'd lived in for years.

Her mother had similar progressive cognitive decline beginning in her early sixties, became severely demented, entered a nursing home, and died when she was about 80. When the patient consulted her physician about her problems, she was told that she had the same problem her mother had had and that there was nothing he could do about it. He wrote "memory problems" in her chart, and therefore the patient was turned down in her application for long-term care.

(continued)

After hearing that she was following in her mother's footsteps and recalling the many years of her mother's decline in a nursing home, she realized there was no treatment and she'd lost the chance to get long-term care insurance. She decided to commit suicide. She called a friend to commiserate, who suggested that she get on a plane and visit. Once she arrived, her friend referred her to a doctor for evaluation.

She began a program very similar to the No More Pills Plan and stuck with most of it. After just 3 months, all of her symptoms had abated: She was able to navigate without problems, remember telephone numbers, prepare reports and do all of her work without difficulty, and read and retain information. Overall, her symptoms vanished. Her memory was now better than it had been in many years. On one occasion, she developed an acute viral illness, discontinued the program, and noticed a decline, which reversed when she reinstated the program. Now, 2½ years later, at age 70, she remains asymptomatic and continues to work full-time.

That's what I call a miraculous success story!

To that end, TCM practitioners don't look at you as a collection of random symptoms. Instead, they look for imbalances in your environment, your diet, your posture, and even in your relationships. They also look for imbalances in your *qi*, your essential energy force, which they believe runs through your body in invisible lines called *meridians*.

The late Robert O. Becker, MD, an orthopedic surgeon and author of *The Body Electric*, dedicated his life to studying and proving that electricity runs through the bodies of humans and animals alike.[50] Although meridians are invisible, through Dr. Becker's work, and that of other researchers, we now know that the actual force that surges through them is very real. Scientific experiments have proven that *qi* is measurable as DC electrical current at exactly the points that TCM refers to as acupuncture meridians.

An Exam Like No Other

The heart of TCM is its reliance on prevention. A TCM practitioner will question you like you've never been questioned by a doctor before; your first examination might last longer than an hour. She will probe deeply into your diet and will examine you more closely than you've ever been examined. Nothing is too small to escape the experienced TCM practitioner's attention. She'll examine your tongue, your pulses, your bowel and urinary habits, your preferred temperature—and don't be offended if you think she's sniffing your breath and body odor, because how you smell gives her clues about your health.

Unlike most Western practitioners, once a TCM healer has sized you up, it's likely that her first recommendation will focus on your diet. She may recommend you practice some tai chi or qigong, both of which are gentle martial arts practices that focus on breath work and balance. She may discuss a course of acupuncture or offer you some Chinese herbs to take home for brewing into tea.

That's not to say that a TCM practitioner won't offer you pills. She very likely might, depending on your problem. But unlike Western pharmaceuticals, which are designed to stamp out symptoms, TCM pills typically contain blends of herbs, which are designed to ease your system back into balance.

As an example of what a difference a different kind of medicine can make, here are two recent studies published in respected Western medical journals.

Advanced breast cancer was the focus of one 2014 study, published in the journal *Cancer*, by a team of researchers from Taipei Medical University, the University of California at San Diego, and the University of Texas School of Public Health. The team scanned the Taiwan National Health Insurance Research Database between 2001 and 2010, looking at cases of women treated for advanced breast cancer with taxanes, a type of chemotherapy drug. They identified 729 women; 115 of them also used traditional Chinese herbal therapy along with the drugs. The researchers reported that the women using TCM along with chemotherapy lived longer than those who used chemo on its own.[51]

In another example, people with impaired glucose tolerance who took the Chinese herbal medicine Tianqi had a 32 percent reduced risk for developing type 2 diabetes compared with a placebo group, reported researchers in a 2014 *Journal of Clinical Endocrinology & Metabolism* article.[52]

What's interesting about studies like these is that, in TCM, you're not simply substituting one (herbal) pill for another (pharmaceutical) pill. The herbs and other medicines in the TCM system are designed to nudge your body gently back to health rather than simply mask symptoms.

Acupuncture 101

Though acupuncture has become more mainstream than ever, with thousands of medical studies proving its benefits for everything from pain conditions to irritable bowel syndrome, some people still consider it at least a little exotic. I use acupuncture for everything from sinusitis to sciatic pain, and rarely if ever have I been disappointed in its results.

One of the most surprising results I've ever had with acupuncture involved a patient who was in her eighties; she had spinal stenosis, a condition in which the spaces in the spine narrow and put pressure on the spinal cord, causing extreme pain. She was in constant pain and also had difficulty walking.

Most doctors would have nothing to offer her, based on her age and the fact that this condition usually gets worse no matter what you do. I suggested acupuncture treatments, and she agreed to come in for twice-weekly visits. At first, the pain relief lasted just a couple of hours after a treatment, but then, her pain-free periods began to lengthen.

After about 7 months of treatment, she was out of pain and walking well. I might have put this down to an exceptional occurrence, but a year or so later, I had the same results with a man in his early nineties who had the same diagnosis.

DR. HOWARD'S NO MORE PILLS RX

1. Ask your doctor about diet, exercise, and supplement options before you agree to take some new drug.

2. If your doctor wants to start you on a brand-new drug, ask if there isn't an older, more tested drug that could be just as effective. If she has nothing to offer, consider finding a health care practitioner who does.

3. Ask your doctor to refer you to a nutritionist/registered dietitian if you need to lose weight.

4. Install a water filter that removes fluoride from your drinking and bath water.

Chapter 2

Immunity Gone Wild

New patients often find their way to me after being disappointed by treatments they've received from other doctors—usually from more than one other doctor. These patients are typically dealing with complex, chronic problems. Perhaps they have digestive difficulties that aren't responding to medication, or they're in chronic pain from sinus problems and headaches, or they're laid low by the pain and fatigue issues that accompany chronic fatigue syndrome or fibromyalgia. They've seen doctor after doctor, taken multiple pharmaceuticals, and endured every lab test in the book, and still they're feeling sick and unhappy.

When I evaluate patients with problems like these, the first thing I do, of course, is ask them what they're eating. And often they'll tell me, "I eat well, Dr. Howard, really! I practically never touch junk food."

Well, that's a start—but just barely. For even if you're eating food that's more or less unprocessed and "healthy," it still might trigger immune system reactions that manifest as various vague, uncomfortable symptoms in sensitive people. One thing I've learned in my 30 years of practice is that these reactions (called immediate- and delayed-type food allergies) are far more widespread than most people realize.

Let's start with immediate-type food allergies first; these are clearly the "attention-getters" of the two. When you have an immediate-type allergic reaction to a certain substance, whether it's peanuts or seafood or bee stings, your body mounts an immediate allergic response as soon as you eat or even touch the offending substance. That response can be life threatening, because your airways can swell and narrow, making breathing difficult or even impossible.

You might suspect that food allergies like these are becoming more prevalent. Think about it: When you were a kid, were peanuts and PB&J sandwiches banned from lunch boxes or playgrounds as they often are now? Did you see labels on food packages warning you about potentially allergenic ingredients or that the product in question was "produced in a facility that also processes nuts, wheat, and other allergens"? Certainly, restaurant menus didn't politely invite you to discuss your "food concerns" with the chef before placing your order.

If you're wondering why more people than ever before have become seriously allergic to many kinds of foods, I hear you—many of my patients do, too. Here's the answer: I believe we're living in an age where our immune systems have become trip-wired to mount assaults against substances that may be (but aren't always) perfectly harmless. That's because there are billions of foreign molecules in our environment that we simply aren't genetically programmed to encounter. (Think about the boatloads of environmental toxins, the Frankenfoods, the oceans of personal care products, the chemicals impregnated into our clothing and upholstery, and the many toxins we use to keep our homes sparkling and pest-free.) It's as if your immune system is in a continual state of high alert; there's always something foreign in the air for it to wave its shield at.

Let's draw a distinction between immediate-type food allergies and delayed-type food allergies. Delayed-type food allergies don't cause the same dramatic, potentially fatal symptoms as do immediate-type food allergies. That's one reason why many doctors sometimes dismiss them as "just sensitivities" rather than the true allergies that they, in fact, are. The reactions delayed-type allergies cause are far subtler and have a slower onset, so they don't occur immediately after you've eaten the offending substance. In fact, you probably won't recognize your symptoms as being food-related, which is why they so often are misdiagnosed as various chronic conditions. Among delayed-type food allergy symptoms are digestive complaints—constipation, diarrhea, gas, heartburn, and bloating. You might have a rash or even eczema. Or you might experience respiratory symptoms, such as wheezing, sinus problems, watery eyes, and headaches. You could even experience migraine headaches or have difficulty concentrating—in fact, you could even suspect you're developing an attention deficit disorder (at your age, of all things).

So with vague but annoying and disconcerting symptoms like these, it's easy to see how your doctor could misdiagnose you with any one of several common problems, from irritable bowel syndrome to sinusitis to gastro-esophageal reflux disease (GERD). And that's where your problems begin, because not only do you not really have the condition—for example, GERD—but now you're being medicated for a condition you don't have with pills you don't need. And many of these pills pose their own insidious side effects.

The No More Pills Food Allergy Quiz

Do you have food allergies? On a scale of 0 to 5 (with 5 being the most), rate how much these symptoms bother you.

1. Abdominal pain ⃝

2. Bloating or swelling (after meals or in the evening) ⃝

3. Belching or passing gas after eating ⃝

4. Frequent bowel movements after eating ⃝

5. Tiredness or falling asleep after eating ⃝

6. Nausea, vomiting ⃝

7. Constipation ⃝

8. Diarrhea ⃝

9. Acid reflux, burning stomach or esophagus ⃝

10. Nasal congestion or discharge ⃝

11. Frequent sinus congestion or infections ⃝

12. Asthma, wheezing, shortness of breath ⃝

13. Frequent mood swings, irritability $\bigcirc$

14. Difficulty concentrating, mental fog $\bigcirc$

15. Hyperactivity, ADD, ADHD $\bigcirc$

16. Anxiety $\bigcirc$

17. Depression $\bigcirc$

18. Memory loss $\bigcirc$

19. Headaches $\bigcirc$

20. Migraines $\bigcirc$

21. Dizziness, loss of balance $\bigcirc$

22. Insomnia $\bigcirc$

23. Muscular pain $\bigcirc$

24. Joint pain or swelling $\bigcirc$

25. Skin rash/eczema/psoriasis $\bigcirc$

Review your results and then check the guide below to learn how likely it is that you have food allergies.

- If you have no symptoms over a 1 or 2 level and a total of eight or fewer symptoms, then you're probably not allergic to foods.
- If you have four, five, or more of these symptoms, even at a 2 or 3 level, you might have food allergies. Try an elimination diet (see page 40) to see if most or all of your symptoms go away.
- If you have levels of 4 or 5 on even two of the symptoms listed, consider looking for a qualified practitioner to test for delayed-type food allergies.
- If you have levels of 4 or 5 on three, four, or especially on five or more of the symptoms listed, get tested as soon as possible.

Immunity 101

To understand how immunity works, let's first take a little crash course in Immunology 101.

The human immune system consists of distinctive cells, tissues, and organs that form a protective force field inside and outside your body to capture, contain, and limit your exposure to harmful viruses, bacteria, and other invaders, including cancer.[1]

It's a very elegant and complicated system, one that should have you marveling at the miraculous way our bodies are designed. The immune system has various components. Let's start with the lymphatic system. This is a network containing vessels, like blood vessels, that carry lymph, the clear fluid that circulates throughout your body, much as blood does. Lymph is your body's cleansing system. It carries out excess tissue fluid, waste material, and immune cells. Along the lymphatic system are thousands (potentially, hundreds of thousands) of lymph nodes.[2] These small, bean-shaped "traps" contain immune cells and are designed to ensnare and dispatch viruses, bacteria, and cancer cells.[3]

The immune system has two highly specialized organs. The spleen makes antibodies, including the IgG antibodies that may attack certain foods you eat. The thymus develops and "programs" T-cells. The immune system also has an important tissue—the marrow—a spongy substance inside the bones. Marrow manufactures many kinds of white blood cells, plus red cells, platelets, and other cells.

Several problems can arise when the immune system isn't working the way it should. Sometimes, often for reasons no one understands, your immune system misdirects its weapons against your own body. When this happens, autoimmune diseases—such as type 1 diabetes, rheumatoid arthritis, or lupus—can arise.

Even more serious problems can arise from a faulty immune system, or one that's temporarily weakened by drugs, such as chemotherapy, or by conditions such as AIDS and severe combined immunodeficiency, the infamous, rare congenital condition that's sometimes called bubble boy disease.[4]

For the purposes of this book, however, we're going to be looking at problems that are far less life threatening, but nonetheless irksome and disruptive. These are the problems caused by an immune system that's attacking your food.

Your Overactive Immune System

There's no way of knowing how many people are unaware that their troublesome symptoms are actually caused by their diets. I can tell you that in my practice, it's a very high percentage. That's because people come to me knowing that I'll help them examine everything in their environments for potential problems. When I do help them remove foods to which they're reactive, we are generally 90 percent successful in taming their symptoms—and most of the time, my patients are utterly stunned (and thrilled, I might add) to discover that what they worried might be some insidious disease actually turned out to be an easily cured delayed-type reaction to certain foods.

Four different types of immune responses exist. There's type I, which we already discussed. It's the body's severe reaction to an allergen. And three other types of allergic responses exist: types II, III, and IV. They're all classified as bona fide types of allergic responses in *Harrison's Principles of Internal Medicine*. I don't know why physicians in the United States focus almost exclusively on type I allergies and pretty much dismiss the others, but that's a standard practice.

However, just because these more subtle and insidious reactions aren't currently recognized in clinical medicine doesn't mean that they don't exist or that they're not extremely harmful. These delayed-type reactions create what I call a slow-burn inflammatory response that can lead to all kinds of health problems—from sinusitis to cancer.

Case in point: People who have a documented sensitivity to gluten have a higher risk of colon cancer if they continue to eat foods that contain gluten. Let's examine these different reactions.

Type I. We call this the immediate-type, because typically the allergic reaction occurs immediately. This reaction is triggered by immunoglobulin E (IgE), which are antibodies produced by the immune system, and mast cells; these release chemicals that cause allergic reactions.[5] You take a bite of, let's say, a peanut, you start to get hives, your lips begin to swell, and your throat begins to close. Time to whip out the EpiPen and get to the ER immediately while you can still breathe.

It's fairly easy to see how this reaction is the one that doctors pay the most attention to—it's immediately life threatening. Testing for type I allergies involves injecting the skin with a small amount of the allergen and observing the response.

Type II. This is a delayed-type response, mediated by immunoglobulin G (IgG). It causes certain types of drug reactions, including reactions to penicillin. It is generally not a common reaction to food.

Type III. This is a delayed-type response, mediated by IgG. However, reactions can occur almost immediately. You've probably seen it yourself—when your skin immediately swells around a vaccine injection site, for example. This is caused by a hypersensitivity response in which antibodies form and inflame the lining of the blood vessels.

The type III response is the most common food-related reaction. Here's what happens: You eat the food—let's say it's dairy. Your body mounts a delayed-type reaction to casein, a food protein in dairy products. Your spleen (remember, it's one of the immune system's organs) clones an army of antibodies keyed to attack the "foreign invader"—in this case, the protein casein. This attack creates a flurry of chemical reactions that irritate the lining of your gut and its blood vessels. As my mentor on this subject, Dr. Francis Murphy, used to say, "These delayed-type food reactions can affect you from head to toe—from migraines to hemorrhoids." Food-related type III responses include bowel symptoms, bloating, headaches, sinus problems, and joint and muscle pain.

Type IV. This is also a delayed-type response. It is mediated by three different types of T cells and can cause contact dermatitis (you might get this if you are allergic to nickel, for example, and wear costume jewelry with nickel in it). It can also cause the tuberculin reaction (the irritation at the site of a skin test for tuberculosis), chronic allergic rhinitis, and chronic asthma. This response is generally more related to skin allergies than to foods.[6,7,8,9]

Here's what often happens: People who have delayed-type allergic responses are tested only for type I reactions and then are told that they're not allergic. What should happen instead? This would be a more accurate way to describe negative responses to type I skin testing—and it's what I'm likely to tell a patient: "Although you don't have type I reactions to this food, you may still be reactive to it." At that point, I would test the patient for IgG reactions to foods and possibly start her on an elimination diet to zero in on what's causing the trouble. And once we identified the food offenders, the patient would eliminate them from her diet.

But that's not what happens for most people. Their doctors tell them they don't test "allergic" to a particular food or foods, so they go right back to eating them, even if they've suspected those foods were causing them problems. And the cycle continues—actually, I should call it a downward spiral. People like these will continue to be misdiagnosed with IBS (irritable bowel syndrome), GERD, eosinophilic esophagitis, or even Crohn's disease. And they will continue to take pills that do nothing to correct their problems—and may even cause problems due to drug side effects.

The "Why" of Food Sensitivities and Intolerances

At least three factors (and potentially more) could be responsible for your reactions to certain foods. In some cases, your body lacks an enzyme that helps break down a compound in a particular food. For example, if you're lactose intolerant, you may have low levels of an enzyme called lactase; when you eat a dairy food like milk or ice cream, you might shortly thereafter experience cramps or even diarrhea because you can't break down the milk sugar, lactose.

Or even more commonly, in the case of dairy, you might have a delayed-type allergic response to the dairy protein, casein. If you are mistakenly told that you're "lactose intolerant," eating dairy foods will still make you sick no matter how much Lactaid you take. That's because you're not reacting to lactose. You're reacting to casein—which the over-the-counter remedy Lactaid can't help you with.

In my opinion, the medical profession is generally pretty casual about the way they refer to dairy food reactions. Many doctors assume that if you react to dairy, you're lactose intolerant, and they'll rarely test you to see whether you're actually reacting to casein.

You could have gluten sensitivity—though you'll test negative for celiac disease (a condition in which your immune system reacts to gluten via damage to the small intestine). However, even though you don't have small intestine damage (yet), you do experience stomach cramps, fatigue, and other symptoms after eating wheat or other gluten-containing foods.

Or you could be reactive to food additives. For example, if your skin flushes or you wheeze or sneeze after drinking wine, you could be sulfite-sensitive. The additive MSG is often a culprit, as are food dyes.

I believe that food additive and environmental pollution reactions are far more widespread than anyone realizes. Just consider how much toxic stuff we're bombarded with on a daily basis. There are the agricultural pesticides on nonorganic vegetables, the chemical additives in processed food, the high-fructose corn syrup, and all the bovine growth hormone, antibiotics, and PCBs in nonorganic milk—and these toxic additives don't even begin to cover the constant assault on our bodies. Rightly, our bodies perceive all these molecules as foreign invaders, so our immune systems are in a constant state of hyperalert.

If you suspect that you are reacting to foods but have gotten negative allergy "scratch tests," I recommend that you find a practitioner to test you for IgG reactions to foods (ELISA testing) or that you go on an elimination diet. It's one of the most effective ways I know to identify which foods are troubling you. Once you know the culprits, simply rid your diet of them. And the good news is, in the next chapter, you'll discover an eating plan that provides delicious, easy meals and snacks that do all the work for you by eliminating most of the troublesome foods. This will go a long way to helping resolve some of your symptoms—and you'll do it without pills!

Is This Our Food—Or a Chemistry Experiment?

All you have to do is read the label on a box of processed food—say, macaroni and cheese or a can of chicken noodle soup or (if the ingredients were listed someplace where you could actually read them) a fast-food meal. That would give you just a clue as to the nearly limitless number of chemical food additives we regularly consume.

The FDA lists hundreds, perhaps thousands, of chemical food additives, and it's virtually impossible to know which of them might pose problems for any individual person.[10] By no means are all of these additives unhealthy; many perform valuable functions, from enhancing color and freshness to providing texture and flavor. The problem is that we really don't know how all these chemicals affect individuals—everyone is different, after all—or whether they might interact with each other to cause reactions in some people. Here are some common food additive categories:

Antioxidants help preserve the shelf life of many foods, particularly those prepared with oils or fats, including bakery products, soup mixes, and sauces.

Emulsifiers, stabilizers, gelling agents, and thickeners keep foods from separating, enable foods to gel, and help add body and thickness.

Flavor enhancers bring out the flavor of foods without imparting one of their own. One of the most controversial of these is monosodium glutamate, or MSG.

Food colors and dyes enhance the way a particular food looks and make it conform better to consumer expectations.

Preservatives allow foods to be kept safely for a longer period of time, and using them is the only method of preservation aside from freezing, canning, or drying that can make a food shelf-stable. Sometimes, preservatives can be simple compounds such as salt, sugar, or vinegar. Chemical preservatives include sulfur dioxide, which stops mold and bacteria growth on dried fruit. Bacon, ham, corned beef, and other cured meats rely on nitrates and nitrites.

Artificial sweeteners, used alone or with sugar, make foods taste sweet—unnaturally so, in my opinion. These include aspartame, saccharin, and sorbitol. See more about these artificial sweeteners on page 67–69.

The No More Pills Elimination Diet

The No More Pills Plan excludes all of the foods known as common allergens. These include:

- Gluten grains (wheat, rye, barley, bulgur, spelt, kamut, triticale, and farro)

- Dairy—cow's, goat's, and sheep's milk products, plus food products that contain dairy in any form

- Corn and all foods that contain corn in any form. You'll need an eagle eye for label reading, as thousands of food products contain corn in some form, including corn-fed beef.

- Soy (again, read labels carefully; soy is often an ingredient in many processed foods)

- Peanuts and other legumes, such as beans, peas, and lentils

- Tree nuts (eliminate only if you have a known allergy)

- All food additives, such as MSG and sulfites (See "Is This Additive Making Me Itch, Wheeze, or Sneeze?" on page 39.)

- Food dyes (FD&C Red, Yellow, Blue, etc.)

- Artificial sweeteners, including aspartame (recently labeled under another alias, "Amino Sweet," also known as NutraSweet and Equal), Splenda, Truvia, saccharin (Sweet'N Low), etc.

Should You Take This Test?

As an alternative to the elimination diet, you might want to consider having an ELISA (enzyme-linked immunosorbent assay) blood test performed. These tests are extremely sensitive and can help quickly pinpoint the foods or additives to which you're reacting. Unlike an elimination diet, however, the tests may be expensive and may not be covered by your insurance.[12]

Start here: Choose a core group of foods that you know don't cause you discomfort. Then every 4 days, add a food. If no symptoms appear, wait 4 days and add another food, such as a serving of pasta. The reason I suggest pasta is that it is made of wheat. If you choose crackers, for example, they could also contain corn products, dyes, or other additives, and if you react to the crackers, you won't know which ingredient causes the problem.

If you do react to the pasta, wait 4 to 5 days until your reaction has completely stopped and add another food, and so on. (*Note:* It's extremely helpful to start a food diary when you begin an elimination diet. Be very detailed: Note the time you eat, what and how much you eat, and every reaction you experience. Keep the diary for a good 2 weeks to establish a pattern of how you're affected by food.)

Fortifying Your Core: My Take on Supplements

I call myself a minimalist when it comes to dietary supplements. I recommend only those that I believe everyone needs to take, even if you eat an excellent, perfectly balanced diet. Nobody needs to take handfuls of supplements to stay well. (This book is titled *No More Pills* for a reason!) And beware any doctor, chiropractor, or "wellness center" that wants to send you off with a shoebox full of pill bottles that you have to buy (from them) every month. The supplements I recommend are truly necessary for health, are made by good companies, are reasonably priced, and can be purchased easily from a store or online. These are my top four.

Probiotics. I recommend that you take a probiotic supplement every day. They improve digestion, immunity, and brain function. In fact, studies have shown that probiotics play a role in improving mood and reducing anxiety—both of which factor into improving a host of chronic diseases.[13] Your gut is an entire ecosystem that only stays in balance if it has plenty of good bacteria, and these days, we simply don't get enough in our diets. Yogurt contains probiotics, but you have to be nonreactive to dairy, and it has to be the plain, organic, unsweetened real stuff, with real organic fruit. Even if you can eat yogurt, I still recommend a daily probiotic supplement.

Because many of my patients are sensitive to dairy, I recommend a dairy-free probiotic supplement. My favorite is Renew Life Ultimate Flora. It is widely available, isn't expensive, and contains a good blend and amount of active bacteria. And you don't have to refrigerate it, as you do with other probiotic supplements. That means you can travel with it, and, better yet, it's easy to remember to take it because it can be on your table instead of in your refrigerator. Take one a day with food.

Fish oil (omega-3 fatty acids). Most Americans don't get enough omega-3s in their diets. We eat too little fish, and we don't eat enough of the healthiest fats, such as walnuts, for example. That's bad news for our brains and our cell membranes, because omega-3s are critical to the way these function. A quick note: Surrounding each cell is a membrane that allows the nutrients to come in and the waste to go out. Unhealthy membranes lead to poor food absorption and inefficient waste removal. And by the way, manufactured fats (trans fats, hydrogenated fats) can penetrate these membranes, and that bad fat sticks around for 120 days—4 months! It's like expecting your cells to function on gunky, dirty old fat—like that in a poorly cleaned deep fryer—instead of using beautifully clear olive oil.

The fish oil brands I recommend are NOW Foods Ultra Omega-3, Nordic Naturals, or Carlson. And make sure that your supplement contains at least 600 milligrams of the EPA/DHA combination. Take one a day with food.

Vitamin D. If you think that this has become the "wonder vitamin," you're right. Most people in the Northern Hemisphere have deficient levels of this vitamin, and because we're careful to use sunscreen when we're in the sun, we no longer get a sufficient amount of vitamin D from being outside. Vitamin D deficiencies are now being linked to a host of chronic illnesses, including diabetes and even depression. A 2014 study links chronic inflammation to low vitamin D levels—and these days, chronic inflammation is linked to most of the chronic diseases I'll cover later in this book. I recommend that people over age 60 take 2,000 IU of vitamin D_3 a day;[14] those younger than 60 need at least 1,000 IU a day. NOW Foods makes a good, inexpensive vitamin D. Take one a day with food.

Vitamin C. Ever since Linus Pauling did his brilliant scientific research on the benefits of vitamin C, it seems as though "medical science" has been trying to discredit it. The minimum daily requirement of vitamin C is 60 milligrams. As far as I'm concerned, this is a pitifully inadequate amount—maybe it's just enough to prevent scurvy or vitamin C deficiency, but certainly not enough to build your collagen and your bones or to keep your immune system functioning at peak levels. There is even some new evidence that a big part of osteoporosis could be vitamin C deficiency.

I recommend at least 500 milligrams a day, and according to Linus Pauling's recommendations, 500 milligrams three to four times a day, with at least 6 to 8 ounces of water, is good. I use NOW Foods Tru-C because it is corn-free, and most corn products now contain unlabeled GMO corn.

● ●

DR. HOWARD'S NO MORE PILLS RX

1. Determine which foods you might be sensitive to via either the elimination diet on page 40 or by getting the ELISA blood test.

2. Once you've learned which foods are posing problems, make sure to ban them from your house. Become a fine-print label reader, and ask what's in your food when dining out. Steer clear of chain and fast-food restaurants, and try to patronize places that put a premium on using fresh, organic, or local foods.

3. Stock your medicine chest with the four essential supplements noted above, and make sure to take them every day.

Chapter 3

The No More Pills Food Plan

Punch the word *diet* into the Amazon.com bookstore and more than 100,000 titles pop up,[1] enough to boggle your strategy of trying to read your way to a healthier, less medicated life. Adding *chronic disease* to *diet* narrows your choices to a staggering 1,900 titles, and many of those books only help you with diets for specific illnesses.[2] So it's quite the challenge to find a diet plan that helps you conquer most, if not all, of the chronic problems that so many of my patients are battling—often more than one condition at once.

That's what sets this book apart. It's about health care, not disease management. What you're about to discover in this chapter is the basic No More Pills Food Plan that you'll need to prevent illnesses such as diabetes, arthritis, IBS, GERD, heart conditions, insomnia, anxiety, allergies, eczema, chronic headaches, migraines, and many others. What's more, you'll learn how to improve these illnesses should you already have them. If your doctor has prescribed pills as the only treatment for a chronic illness, then this book is for you.

Later in the book, in sections that cover each condition separately, you'll learn how certain foods, gentle activities (think walking and yoga), mind-body exercises, herbs, and other natural solutions are scientifically proven to improve the conditions that trouble you most. Who knows? You may be able to put down those pills forever—or at the very least, take fewer of them.

What Your Doctor Can't Tell You

I was searching through my records to find a patient who'd be an excellent example of my overall approach to helping people lessen their dependence on medications, and guess what? It turned out to be me. So what kind of health problems could a doctor like me have, what with all my knowledge about disease prevention and healthy eating? Good question.

Turns out, some challenges come courtesy of your genes, and in my case, I inherited something called polycystic ovary syndrome (PCOS) from my mother (her sister also had the condition). PCOS produces higher estrogen levels and insulin resistance, and it predisposes women who have it to infertility, diabetes, and hypothyroidism, among other things. Happily, I was able to take hormone treatments and gave birth to two wonderful children. I think the treatments and the births probably put me into remission. The only problem I dealt with was a tendency to have low blood sugar if I didn't eat often enough. I was fine through menopause (a time when problems often crop up), but then I broke my foot in a freak accident. I blamed my unwilling but necessary inactivity for the fact that in 2 years, little by little, I gained more than 20 pounds. Then my blood sugar started to creep up, too—into the triple digits, high enough to be worrisome.

That was enough for me. I was scared. As a doctor, I knew just how much damage high blood sugar could do—think of it as having a tiny battering ram inside your most fragile blood vessels, slamming, "denting," and weakening blood vessel walls. And that's just for starters.

I thought about the pills I'd have to take, and I even put myself on a popular diabetes medication for a few weeks and started on a diet. But then I thought, "What am I doing?" I'd never let one of my patients go down this route. I had to let go of my fears and follow my own best advice.

I'd heard about the popular Paleo diet, which eliminates grains, sugar, dairy, legumes, and alcohol. What attracted me wasn't the notion of eating like a cave person—modern humans have indeed evolved considerably since that long-ago time. What compelled me to give it a try was the science behind it (more about that later).

I added some interval exercise work because science showed interval training could reduce fasting blood sugar and A1C, a measure of blood sugar taken over time. Instead of sugary snacks, I added nuts—especially pistachios, which studies show can lower blood sugar. And I took the blood sugar–lowering natural supplements I recommend to patients: berberine and bitter melon. In just 4 months, I'd lost 24 pounds, and my blood sugar was—and still is—normal. Best of all, no more pills!

Here's another example that illustrates why this book will be so helpful to you. A 60-year-old acquaintance of mine—let's call her Christine—recently told me about her visit to her new primary care doctor. Though she looked the very picture of good health and had the energy of a much younger woman, Christine was taking pills to control her type 2 diabetes, her high blood pressure, and her high cholesterol.

Her new doctor reviewed her history, asked her how she was feeling, listened to her chest, took her blood pressure, scheduled her for a blood test, and told her to have her pharmacy phone the doctor's office when she needed refills for her meds. That office visit lasted less than 15 minutes.

It should go without saying that 15 minutes is hardly enough time to assess a new patient's needs. And, of course, I wished that my pal had questioned her new doctor more closely about other tools she could use to address her chronic conditions (the very tools you'll learn about in this book). But I understand how it goes. Even if you're not afraid that the doctor won't answer your questions (and sadly, some doctors do make you afraid—very afraid), it may be that you feel she's incredibly busy, she doesn't have time, and that maybe your concerns are trivial compared to those of her other patients. After all, the doctor has really sick people to take care of, and you're grateful you're not one of them.

What I really wish for Christine, and the millions like her, is that her doctor would have helped her change up her habits so that she could get off her medications or at least lower her dosages. Doctors can be instrumental in this by helping people adjust their diets so that they can dial down inflammation, lessen the chances that they're having delayed-type allergic reactions to foods, and improve their overall digestion, for starters. But finding a doctor who can discuss the fine points of optimizing your nutrition isn't always so easy.

As I mentioned previously, don't forget that most doctors are ill-equipped to give you the nutritional advice you really need. The lack of nutritional education in medical schools is appalling, considering that obesity and all the terrible chronic diseases it promotes are our number one public health problem.

Medical Schools: Nutritionally Challenged

Here's a great illustration: Back in 1995, Robert F. Kushner, MD, professor in medicine at Northwestern University Feinberg School of Medicine in Chicago, conducted a survey of more than 2,000 primary care physicians across the United States. He was hoping to find out how many of them actually delivered nutrition counseling to their patients. Here's what he learned: More than two-thirds of the doctors provided counseling to less than 40 percent of their patients, and those who did offer nutritional advice spent less than 5 minutes discussing dietary changes. Yet, nearly 75 percent of doctors surveyed said that they believe the physician is responsible for providing nutrition counseling to patients—and that doing so is important.[3]

As a result of his study, Dr. Kushner called for action: He suggested a comprehensive approach designed to change physicians' counseling practices.[4] But even after this and other major initiatives, like Healthy People 2010, a government program that encouraged people to improve their health,[5] not much progress has been made.

"The prevailing belief today is that little has changed," wrote Kathryn M. Kolasa, PhD, RD, professor of nutrition in the department of family medicine at East Carolina University in Greenville, North Carolina, in a 2010 paper in *Nutrition in Clinical Practice*. But it has—a little. It's gotten *worse*. Even *fewer* doctors were offering nutritional advice in 2010 than in 1995, according to Dr. Kolasa's study.[6]

I'm among the minority of medical doctors who focus on nutrition and who make sure patients get the right eating plan for their needs. But you don't have to fly to Chicago and see me to get this level of nutritional advice and personal attention—you're holding it in your hand. Let's plan a diet for you that will, in just a month or so, make you feel better than you have in years.

What Is the No More Pills Plan?

For the last 30 years, I've been counseling my patients about the ways proper nutrition can help improve their health conditions. The famous (if mistranslated) Hippocrates quote "Let food be thy medicine, and medicine be thy food" is a favorite of mine.[7] Another favorite is more recent, from the philosopher Wendell Berry, who's the 2010 recipient of the National Humanities Medal. He said, "People are fed by the food industry, which pays no attention to health, and are treated by the health industry, which pays no attention to food."

The key benefit of the No More Pills Plan is that it reduces body-wide inflammation. That's what I designed it to do, and that's why I'm so committed to it. It's a revolutionary way to help you heal. We now understand that inflammation sets the stage for a host of—if not most—chronic diseases. What's more, my plan is built on foods that cause virtually no delayed-type allergies in most people. Because the plan is extremely low in carbohydrates and emphasizes foods that are low on the glycemic index (more about that later), it naturally balances blood sugar and doesn't leave you victim to the kinds of blood sugar spikes and dips that affect your mood and your energy.

The plan focuses on pure, whole foods and is free of gluten and grains. It emphasizes organic, non-GMO vegetables and lean, natural proteins, such as wild fish, grass-fed and organic meats and poultry, organic eggs, and nuts and seeds. You can enjoy good-for-you fats and small amounts of honey or organic maple syrup. Plus, you can have what some of us still think of as the three major food groups: coffee, wine, and chocolate! All of these wonderful ingredients lend themselves perfectly to delectable, family-pleasing, and easy-to-make recipes (you'll find them starting on page 255). In fact, when I think about the No More Pills Plan, I don't think deprivation and hunger; I think of fun eating and plenty of scrumptious food.

You could say that the No More Pills Plan is my variation on a Paleo-style diet, with the addition of many Mediterranean-style dishes. But I'd rather that you consider the No More Pills Plan simply as a way of eating that improves your health naturally. You'll chill out inflammation; your symptoms will ease; and as a bonus, you'll probably lose some weight—without even trying! The No More Pills Plan is the culmination of what I've learned about nutrition throughout my 3 decades of medical practice. I believe it's the perfect way to eat (in fact, it's how I eat every day!), and it can help you reduce, or get off, the medications you're taking.

In general (though you won't be counting!), the No More Pills Plan will consist of 30 to 40 percent healthy fats, 30 to 40 percent protein, and 10 to 20 percent carbs.

The No More Pills Plan Benefits

This plan offers a satisfying and delectable way to eat, and many of the benefits of the No More Pills Plan are scientifically proven. Remember, even though I didn't design the plan primarily as a weight loss diet, I lost 25 pounds on this diet without even trying, and I never had to count calories or feel hungry. Almost all of my patients who've tried it have also lost a substantial amount of weight. And that's a clear bonus because carrying too many pounds contributes to most of the chronic conditions that people take pills in hopes of correcting. Here are some of the key features that make the No More Pills Plan so successful.

Increased protein. Organic, grass-fed, and naturally lean meat; wild and organically farmed seafood; and organic eggs from free-range chickens will make up about 30 to 40 percent of your diet. Diets high in protein are proven to make you feel fuller and more satisfied and to help you burn calories more efficiently. What's more, a 2008 study suggested that high-protein diets can also improve heart disease risk factors.[8]

Low carbs. The No More Pills Plan is free of grains and gluten, plus it's extremely low in sugar. Those aspects of the plan slash the amount of simple carbs you'll be eating, which are responsible for spiking blood sugar. How does this help you lose the pills? A major 2014 study, published in the *Annals of Internal Medicine,* concluded that low-carb diets effectively lower your risk for heart disease. What's more, said the researchers, low-carb diets beat low-fat diets for helping you lose weight. On this plan, you'll be eating lots of nonstarchy vegetables and low-glycemic fruits, which are low in carbohydrates and loaded with nutrients.[9]

High fiber. You might worry about whether you're getting enough fiber once you purge your diet of cereals, breads, and other grain- and gluten-containing foods. Rest easy—you'll be getting plenty of fiber on the No More Pills Plan. The vegetables you'll be eating—including various members of the squash family, leafy greens, and green veggies—and fruits, such as apples and pears, will provide more than enough fiber to keep you healthy. Recent research has linked high-fiber diets, by the way, to a lower risk of heart disease. In fact, researchers who pored over 22 studies published between 1990 and 2013 reported that the more fiber in your diet, the lower your chances for having a heart attack.[10]

More and better fats. Remember the days when we were told that slashing fat from our diets was a smart health move? Well, as we know now, that was simply terrible advice. In fact, when the food industry jumped on that bandwagon, the packaged foods they pushed as "low fat" usually replaced the fat with lots of sugar, salt, and other unhealthy ingredients. In the end, going "low fat" made us gain more weight and also upped our risks for diabetes, heart disease, and other illnesses. Now we know better—and that's why the No More Pills Plan, like the healthful and scientifically proven Mediterranean diet, contains up to 50 percent healthy fats. I'm talking about omega-3 fats. Some omega-3s, called EPA and DHA, are found in flaxseed, walnuts, sardines, and wild salmon. Another type, ALA, comes from Brussels sprouts, kale, spinach, and salad greens. We know through research that omega-3s protect against heart disease; newer studies suggest they may also help protect against cancers, inflammatory bowel disease, and autoimmune conditions like rheumatoid arthritis.[11] What's more, the grass-fed, organic meats you'll enjoy on this plan contain a fat called conjugated linoleic acid, or CLA, which helps reduce body fat and increases lean body mass.[12]

No starchy grains. The No More Pills Plan strips a whole layer (that would be the grains) off the bottom of the old food pyramid, just as it strips a whole layer (or layers!) of fat off the bottom (and top) of your body. This is a long overdue change in the way we eat. I'm convinced that the low-fat, high-carb diets that were once so popular have helped create the epidemics of obesity, diabetes, and Alzheimer's disease we face today.

Nutrient-dense, not calorie-dense. How does this aspect of the food plan help you get off pills? Some of the conditions you take pills for are actually caused by vitamin or mineral deficiencies, and your prescription drugs do nothing to change that. In fact, in a landmark study published in the *Journal of the American Medical Association,* deficiencies of several key nutrients, including D, E, and B vitamins, were linked to several diseases, including colorectal, prostate, and breast cancer; heart disease; osteoporosis; and bone loss. The No More Pills Plan delivers nutrient-rich foods to ensure that your vitamin needs are met. For some conditions, I recommend taking vitamin supplements (see Part II). Since so many people living in North America have vitamin D deficiencies, I recommend that most people under 60 supplement with 1,000 IU of vitamin D daily.[13] People over 60 should take 2,000 IU daily.

Anti-inflammatory. Chronic, body-wide inflammation is often mentioned these days as a cause of many illnesses. But here's the real truth: Inflammation is not a "cause" of illness. Something else (for example, allergies to foods or chronic infection) causes the inflammation—and the illness. In fact, I have had two food allergic patients in their forties who have actually had strokes at their young age. It turns out they were both reactive to gluten. In addition to inflammation in their gut lining, their reactions to gluten actually inflamed the lining (endothelium) of their blood vessels. Now that both are on gluten-free diets, they've recovered from their strokes and are happily healthy.

The Benefits of a Low-GI Diet

In this case, *GI* doesn't mean gastrointestinal, if you were wondering. It stands for *glycemic index.* You've probably read about eating foods that rank low on the glycemic index, but you may not know exactly what that means or why it's so healthy. A key aspect of the No More Pills Plan is that it focuses on low-glycemic foods.

The glycemic index, developed by researchers at the University of Sydney in Australia, is a ranking of carbohydrates on a scale of 0 to 100 based on how high a food raises your blood sugar levels after you eat it. Foods with a high GI value are absorbed rapidly and quickly affect your blood sugar—something that is absolutely *not* what we want when you're following the No More Pills Plan.

Foods with a low GI value are more slowly digested and absorbed, so blood sugar and insulin levels rise slowly. Research from the Harvard School of Public Health clearly links higher risks for type 2 diabetes and heart disease to diets with higher GI levels. To find out what a particular food's GI value is, visit glycemicindex.com, the Web site that the University of Sydney maintains and updates listing the GI values of foods.[14]

The No More Pills Position on Gluten

You'd have to be living in an alternate universe not to have heard about the great gluten controversy. Gluten-free diets are considered by many to be the new diet fetish of the 21st century. The food industry has jumped on the bandwagon, offering countless gluten-free products (and it always tickles me to see a gluten-free label slapped on a product that never previously contained the stuff). But there's robust science behind all the reasons to be gluten-free.

Unlike sketchy diet fads of the past (the Scarsdale diet comes to mind), the No More Pills Plan has some pretty astonishing health benefits—and a big part of its effectiveness is because it's a grain-free diet. Even if you've seen the headlines and read the stories, you may still not understand why nutritionally astute doctors like me advise that you avoid all foods that contain gluten.

What Is Gluten?

What do you think of when you hear the word *gluten*? These days, you probably think it's that stuff so many people seem to be eliminating from their diets, and you're probably at least a little unclear as to what the hoopla is all about. Gluten is actually a sticky protein that holds bread products together and provides their chewiness. Although almost 200 proteins are members of the gluten family, gluten is most often thought of as a composite of just two proteins, glutenin and gliadin, found in wheat as well as rye, barley and oats, bulgur, couscous, kamut, semolina, spelt, triticale, and other grains.[15]

In addition to the gluten grains listed above, many other foods contain gluten, especially processed and packaged foods. Happily, your No More Pills Plan doesn't include processed, junk, fast, or packaged foods, so no worries about running into the hidden gluten in those products.[16]

As discussed in Chapter 2, your body can have delayed-type allergic reactions to many food proteins, including gluten. (Another problem food protein for many people is casein, found in milk.) Food intolerances to substances such as gluten arise when your body has trouble processing certain components of a food, writes Amy C. Brown, PhD, a registered dietitian and researcher at the University of Hawaii in Honolulu, in a study published in a gastroenterology journal in 2012.[17]

Until 2008, most physicians considered only one response to gluten to be worth consideration—the very serious health problem known as celiac disease.[18] Celiac disease is caused by a gluten allergy that actually triggers lesions and other intestinal damage. But when a gold standard study showed that people with irritable bowel syndrome (IBS) who did *not* have celiac disease experienced IBS symptom relief after following a gluten-free diet, quite a number of us in the medical profession realized that at least some people without celiac disease could absolutely benefit from going on a gluten-free diet.[19]

Experts estimate that 1 in 200 people suffers from celiac disease. But David Perlmutter, MD, a neurologist and author of the book *Grain Brain*, begs to differ with that estimate. He believes the number is closer to 1 in 30 because many people with celiac disease simply have yet to be diagnosed.[20]

He—and others—insist that a host of gluten health problems exist beyond celiac disease, and I agree because such problems crop up among my patients time and time again. Many of my patients, for example, have been tested for celiac disease in the hope of finding a reason (and solution) for their disturbing digestive complaints. When the celiac test results have come back negative, doctors have treated (and medicated) those patients for other conditions, such as IBS or GERD. But their cramps, bloating, diarrhea, constipation, heartburn, gas, and other symptoms usually don't go away. And that's often when patients look to me or another like-minded doctor for help.

The fact is that gluten can cause many people to have difficult digestive issues even if they don't have celiac disease. What's more, gluten reactions can cause problems that go beyond the gut, says Dr. Perlmutter in his book. After all, he's a board-certified neurologist. People don't bring their digestive complaints to him; they come in for neurological problems. He asserts that these delayed-type gluten allergies can involve any organ in the body—including the brain.[21] I'm acutely aware of this problem, too, and have treated people with gluten problems for more than 30 years. Recently, others have discovered that both he and I are correct. Turns out, gluten can be responsible for a variety of neurological problems, such as peripheral neuropathy, a painful condition affecting the nerves, says a 2010 paper published in the journal *Lancet*.[22] And a link between migraines and other chronic headaches triggered by gluten and dairy sensitivities was uncovered in research Dr. Perlmutter himself published in the journal *Integrative Medicine* in 2013.[23]

Based on what I hear from colleagues, and from what I see in my own patients, I believe that gluten sensitivity rates are rising and that more and more people are having delayed-type allergic reactions to foods containing gluten. One researcher has estimated that for every person with celiac disease, at least six or seven people have gluten sensitivity.[24] I bet it's even more than that.

What on earth could be causing the problem? After all, traditionally, we think of wheat as "the staff of life," as an essential food that goes way back to Biblical times. How many of us actually pray, "Give us this day our daily bread"? Certainly, before the industrialization of agriculture, wheat *was* a staff of life. But since then, we've managed to manipulate the living daylights out of wheat so that growers can have bigger crops and make more money. Also, they've bred wheat so that it can be baked into the breads Americans have come to prefer—soft, squishy, and white.

Plant breeding has actually made wheat gluten "stronger" over time. As a result, today's wheat produces bread dough that has more volume, so it bakes into more loaves—making bread and other bakery products cheaper to produce.[25] Some researchers suggest that the genetic engineering of wheat may lead to more people becoming sensitive to gluten.

What's more, bread, pasta, and other grain products aren't the only gluten-containing foods. Gluten is now a food additive that shows up in soups, sauces, potato chips, meat products, ice cream, and even candies. What's more, gluten is sometimes added to pills and dietary supplements— providing yet another reason to become a sharp-eyed label reader.[26] And finally, additives and pesticide residues in wheat products can make them much more allergenic.

The Benefits of Being Dairy-Free

"Milk: It Does a Body Good" and "Got Milk?" are two of the most enduring and memorable advertising taglines of all time. Which was exactly the point of the dairy industry's gazillion-dollar campaigns to get Americans to drink more milk. Just recently, the industry invested in a new $50 million campaign to replace "Got milk?" Their new hook? "Milk Life."[27, 28]

I'm sorry to hear that. Personally, when it comes to improving our nutrition, I can think of far better ways to spend $50 million than on an advertising campaign. And I'm sorry to burst your bubble if you're among the majority of people who think of dairy products as healthy foods. In fact, for most people, they are anything but.

Let's do some dairy foods myth-busting. When I discuss dairy products with my patients and suggest that, for most of them, it's best to remove the white stuff from their diets, the first reaction is usually, "But what about my calcium and bone strength? Isn't milk essential for that?"

Actually, it's not, according to some scientific studies. While it's true that calcium is a key bone-building mineral, dairy products may not be as useful a calcium source as we've been led to believe. "Clinical research shows that dairy products have little or no benefit for bones," states the Physicians Committee for Responsible Medicine (PCRM), a nonprofit organization that supports bringing nutrition into medical education and practice. The organization cites the famous Harvard Nurses' Health Study, which followed 72,000 women for 18 years. It showed "no protective effect of increased milk consumption on fracture risk."[29] And though we think of milk as a key part of our children's diets, the PCRM points to two studies: one, published in *Pediatrics* in 2005, showed that milk consumption did not improve bone integrity in children; and a 2012 paper in the *Archives of Pediatrics & Adolescent Medicine* that suggested consuming dairy products didn't prevent stress fractures in adolescent girls, after tracking their diets, activity, and incidence of stress fractures over 7 years.[30]

Further, it's clear that many people are actually allergic to dairy products. Eat a bowl of ice cream or down a glass of milk, and you might suddenly experience some very uncomfortable digestive complaints.

Two separate issues are involved when we're talking about the problems dairy products cause. One is lactose intolerance; another is an allergy to casein, which is a protein found in dairy products.

One of my saddest doctor abuse stories concerns lactose intolerance versus casein allergy. One of my patients came in—in tears—to tell me her experience. She'd complained about her digestive problems to her doctor, telling him it happened mostly when she ate dairy. The doctor asked, gruffly, "Don't you know about lactose intolerance?" Then he went stalking out of the room, only to return in a minute with packets of Lactaid pills. He slapped them down in front of her and ordered her to take them.

Now, understand that Dr. Abusive didn't bother to take any further medical history, nor did he attempt to test whether she was actually reacting to casein, lactose, or both. Turns out, when I tested her, she proved to be allergic to casein.

Just leave it to us to explain the difference. And here's the punch line—if your reaction to dairy involves a delayed-type allergy to casein, the milk protein, then Lactaid, a product containing the enzyme that breaks down lactose, the milk sugar, will do you absolutely no good.

Here's why: When we eat or drink dairy products, we ingest lactose, a sugar found in all dairy products. To digest it, the small intestine secretes an enzyme called lactase. It breaks lactose into the sugars glucose and galactose, which are then absorbed into the bloodstream.

If you have "lactose intolerance," you'll experience uncomfortable diarrhea, cramps, bloating, and gas after you've downed a glass of milk or scooped down some ice cream.[31] But many people whose doctors have told them that they are lactose intolerant are actually casein allergic. Based on the doc's advice, however, they go to the drugstore, pick up some Lactaid, and try to eat or drink dairy products. And still they get sick. Why?

The answer is that casein can cause a type III allergic reaction (see "Your Overactive Immune System" on page 35). When your immune system mistakes casein for a harmful invader, it will produce those allergy (IgG) antibodies we talked about in Chapter 2, which are present in the delayed-type response. Your symptoms could appear as digestive symptoms, like diarrhea, gas, or bloating, or as congestive symptoms, such as sinus congestion, headaches, and coughing. Whatever reaction you experience, your doctor could mistakenly medicate you for whatever he thinks is wrong with you and be oblivious to the fact that dairy foods are the culprit. Over time, the damage a casein allergy causes to your gut can wreak havoc with your digestion and can leave you prone to all kinds of problems. How can you be sure? Try an elimination diet like the No More Pills Plan or ask for the ELISA test. Either of these can help determine whether or not you have a delayed-type allergy to the casein in dairy products.

Even if you're not allergic or intolerant, I still don't recommend that you include dairy foods while following this plan.

Organic Is Best

The weight of the evidence is in: Organically grown and raised fruits, vegetables, meats, and fish are better for us than those sprayed with pesticides or fed pesticide-laced grain. To me, this issue has always been a no-brainer: How could spraying poison on food and then eating it be a good thing for the human body? And as far as genetically modified (GMO) produce is concerned, I'm firmly on the side of something called the precautionary principle (see "The Precautionary Principle" on page 60). These aren't the only reasons why the No More Pills Plan relies solely on organically grown produce and protein.

I, and many like-minded health care practitioners, firmly believe that the proliferation of toxic chemicals, such as pesticides, in our environment is linked to the rise in numbers of people whose immune systems are overreacting to once harmless foods. When so many foreign chemicals bombard us, it puts our immune systems on "overdrive" and makes our bodies more likely to react unpredictably. And another thing: As far as I'm concerned, the industry of making and transporting toxic chemicals poses knowable and unknowable risks to our public health and safety. Going organic on a massive scale would lessen our dependence on these poisons—and that, I believe, could have an enormous and positive impact on our health and that of our planet.

Here's what we know about the health impacts of pesticides.[32]

- Exposures to pesticides (more than 17,000 are currently on the market) have been linked to brain and central nervous system disruption, infertility, a multitude of cancers, and even changes to our DNA.

- Children born to mothers who lived near pesticide-treated fields are six times more likely to be autistic.

- Switching to an organic diet for just 5 days virtually eliminates any signs of exposure to organophosphate pesticides among school-age children.

- A nationwide study found elevated risk for several types of childhood cancers for children living near fields treated with pesticides.

- More than 80,000 synthetic chemicals are used in this country, but only a few hundred have been tested for safety.

I recommend that you look for the green and white USDA Organic label on all the foods you buy. Right now, that label stands for farmers, ranchers, and food processors who sell products following a defined set of standards to produce organic foods. According to the USDA, these standards cover the product from farm to table, including soil and water quality, pest control, livestock practices, and rules for food additives.[33]

The No More Pills Food List

Consider making two copies of this list. Keep one handy in your kitchen, and take the other with you when you shop. It's your essential guide to the No More Pills Plan.

Enjoy

- Grass-fed organic meats (including game), organic chicken, wild-caught or organically farmed fish and seafood, and organic eggs.

- Fresh organic fruits. Choose fruits with lower fruit sugar content and higher fiber content, such as berries, apples, pears, or peaches. High-fiber fruits have the least impact on raising your blood sugar. Eat tropical fruits and watermelon very sparingly or avoid them, because their sugar content is much higher.

- Fresh or frozen organic vegetables—all veggies except peas are on the list. Enjoy these starchy vegetables: sweet potatoes, yams, and the many different squash varieties. (Spaghetti squash makes a satisfying pasta substitute!)

- Nuts and seeds (not peanuts, which are legumes).

- Healthy oils: cold-pressed organic olive, coconut, sesame, sunflower, walnut, macadamia, and avocado.

- Small amounts of local honey or 100 percent pure, preferably organic, maple syrup.

- Pure stevia as a sweetener (not blends such as Truvia). SweetLeaf and Pyure are good brands.

Enjoy Occasionally

- Once or twice a week, enjoy one small potato or half of a larger one—preferably with blue, purple, or golden flesh and eaten with its skin.[34]

- Two or three servings a week (organic only) of quinoa or wild rice, as long as you maintain a weight that's healthy for you.

- Two to three glasses of organic, nonsulfited wine per week with food.

- One or two squares of dark chocolate two or three times a week. Buy fair-trade organic chocolate bars. Look for higher percentages of cacao—more than 70 is best—and make sure to choose the brands lowest in sugar.

The Obesity–Food Chemical Connection

If you're still looking for motivation to choose foods free of chemical food additives (no organic food can contain these potentially toxic substances, by the way), here's some ammo. In 2012, researchers from the Innsbruck Medical University in Austria discovered a potential link between two food additives and weight gain. In their test-tube study, they learned that sodium sulphite and sodium benzoate appear to delay the release of the hormone leptin. The hormone's job is to tell you that you're full. Based on this study, it's entirely conceivable that eating these additives in processed foods could make feeling full an elusive sensation—thus making overeating (and becoming overweight) more likely.[35]

Researchers are also studying whether or not synthetic environmental contaminants could be contributing to the global obesity epidemic, according to a 2014 report in the journal *Current Obesity Reports*. Though the evidence isn't yet solid, the authors suggest that many contaminants do interfere with our endocrine function, insulin signaling, and the way our fat cells behave. But the fact is, we still haven't studied the effects of the combination of intentional food additives (such as artificial sweeteners, colors, and emulsifiers) and unintentional compounds (think pesticides, for example) on human metabolism.[36] We just don't know what the health consequences of combining these compounds might be, especially years down the road.

And that's another excellent reason, if you ask me, to live by the precautionary principle. Until we know for a fact that these additives don't impact us in a negative way, why not go organic and avoid them?

Avoid

- Cereal grains. For example, avoid wheat, rye, barley, oats, spelt, millet, corn, buckwheat, and white or brown rice (in addition to the gluten sources mentioned earlier under "What Is Gluten?" on page 52).
- Legumes. All beans, peas, and peanuts.
- All dairy products from cows, goats, and sheep, including milk, yogurt, and cheese. Also avoid foods that contain dairy in any form.
- Refined or raw sugars, including cane and corn sugars, and refined maple sugar.
- Refined oils, hydrogenated or partially hydrogenated oils, trans fats, and any foods made with these unhealthy fats, including grain, bean, or seed oils, such as soybean, cottonseed, sunflower, grapeseed, corn, safflower, and canola.

The Precautionary Principle

In a nutshell, this principle holds that we already have good scientific evidence and shouldn't wait for more to come in before we act cautiously about products or technologies that potentially could affect our health or the health of our planet. To me, it's a reaffirmation of the Hippocratic Oath I took when I began my medical practice—"First, do no harm." Here's an example: For decades, we had strong reasons to believe that smoking tobacco was terribly unhealthy. And happily, that was enough to persuade millions of people to stop smoking, well before all of the scientific evidence was finally in and publicly made available (despite the tobacco companies' extensive efforts *not* to make the information public; instead, they countered it with sexy advertising). The quitters, wisely, were employing the precautionary principle. Unfortunately, many thousands of smokers still believe the science isn't fully established or are unwilling to believe it (or are so addicted they can't quit) and so continue to smoke. As a result, many thousands develop lung cancer or other serious health problems.[37]

- Processed foods, food additives, artificial sweeteners and flavorings, food dyes, and excess salt.
- All fast and junk foods.[38, 39]
- Sugary drinks, including natural fruit juice and soft drinks.

Herbs and Spices

Aromatic and flavor-rich herbs and spices are key additions to the foods you'll enjoy on the No More Pills Plan. Not only do they add a savory shot to everything you eat, but many also offer significant phytochemicals that, together with foods, can deal a blow to chronic diseases. Make sure to add fresh or dried organic herbs and spices to everything you cook, and the recipes in Part III are a great way to start. Try these delectable herbs and spices for starters—and experiment with plenty of others.

Parsley. Two tablespoons of fresh parsley provides more than 150 percent of your daily requirement for vitamin K, which is essential for healthy blood and bones.

Oregano. If you use only one herb in your cooking, make it oregano. This potent herb (which some chefs think actually tastes better dried) contains, on average, up to 20 times more cancer-fighting antioxidants than other herbs. It even holds its own against fruit: According to USDA researchers, 1 tablespoon of fresh oregano has the antioxidant potency of an entire apple. Gram for gram, the herb has twice the antioxidant activity of blueberries.

Rosemary. This herb can actually boost your performance on speed and accuracy tests, says a study from Northumbria University in the United Kingdom. Plus, researchers from the University of Arkansas, Iowa State University, and Kansas State University found that cooking meats with rosemary can reduce the carcinogenic compounds that form when cooking over high heat, like on a barbecue or grill.

Turmeric. An antioxidant ingredient, curcumin, is what gives turmeric (often used in curries) its yellow color. Research has already linked this super ingredient to a reduced risk of type 2 diabetes and Alzheimer's disease. And a study in the journal *Gastroenterology* found that it may help ward off tumors associated with colon cancer.

Ginger. Studies show that this spicy rhizome can soothe stomachaches, aid circulation, suppress nausea (it's especially good for easing motion sickness), decrease blood pressure, and curb arthritis pain. Plus, it may even reduce your cancer risk.

Cinnamon. In a study of people with type 2 diabetes, German researchers found that cinnamon can reduce blood sugar levels by 10 percent, possibly because compounds in cinnamon activate enzymes that stimulate insulin receptors. The sweet spice has also been shown to help lower levels of cholesterol and triglycerides, blood fats that may contribute to diabetes risk.[40]

Garlic. People who consumed lots of garlic had lower rates of ovarian, colorectal, and other cancers, says a research review in the *American Journal of Clinical Nutrition*. Garlic contains more than 70 active phytochemicals, including allicin, which many studies have shown decreases high blood pressure by as much as 30 points. Garlic may help prevent strokes as well by slowing arterial blockages, according to a yearlong clinical study at UCLA. It's best to chop or crush fresh garlic and let it stand for 10 minutes—that way, its cardiovascular and cancer-fighting benefits will withstand cooking.[41]

Drink for Your Health

So now that you have an excellent foundation for how to eat your way to better health (and, hopefully, to a life dominated by fewer pills), let's turn our attention to the liquid portion of the No More Pills Plan. Drinking the right kinds of fluids will be essential to your success, and, as you'll discover, some liquids are clearly superior to others—in fact, some drinks do a fantastic job at helping you down the path to taking fewer pills. On the other hand, others are totally off-limits in the No More Pills Plan—including one class of beverages that could actually sabotage your progress.

Water

You can't drive a car unless it's topped off with the right kind of oil, and that's a pretty good way to illustrate your body's need for water. Plenty of water not only keeps all of your fluid levels in balance, but it also plays a key role in so many of the processes that keep you alive—including metabolism, breathing, sweating, waste removal, body temperature regulation, and cushioning bones and joints, among many other actions.

Our Watery Bodies

It's easy to understand why drinking enough water is essential for good health, once you realize how much water our organs contain.[42]

Adult human body	60 percent H_2O
Lungs	83 percent H_2O
Bones	31 percent H_2O
Brain and heart	73 percent H_2O
Muscles and kidneys	79 percent H_2O

How much water you need to drink every day has been debated, but I believe something like 48 to 64 ounces of water or other fluids (from the list that follows) is a good amount to shoot for.

I have concerns about chemicals in our water system, which is why I recommend that you use a water filter in your home to make sure you're drinking water that's free of harmful toxins. You can find affordable and effective brands—see page 15 for details.

If water's just too ho-hum for you, you can zap it up by adding citrus slices, crushed fresh herbs (I love mint and lemon balm), or even slices of cucumber. If you add lemon, lime, or cucumber slices, scrub the outside of the lemons or limes with an ecofriendly detergent and rinse them well, and wash and peel the cucumber. You can also enjoy any of the sparkling waters (not sweetened or artificially sweetened) that come in so many flavors these days.[43]

Green Tea

Hands down, green tea is one of the most health-giving beverages on the planet. Made from the unfermented leaves of the tea plant (*Camellia sinensis*), it's packed with potent antioxidants called polyphenols. Tea's polyphenols are classed as catechins, and green tea contains six different catechin compounds, the most studied and active of which is epigallocatechin gallate (EGCG). Green tea also contains stimulants, including caffeine, theobromine, and theophylline. And in one of those wonders of nature in which a plant's medicinal compounds actually balance each other out, green tea also contains L-theanine, an amino acid that has been studied for its calming effects. Study after study has confirmed green tea's many benefits, so let's take a look at what this delicate quaff has to offer.

Protects your heart. Though they're not sure why, researchers who study green tea estimate that drinking three cups a day can lower your heart attack risk by 11 percent. It also might help lower blood pressure, especially in older people whose blood pressure drops after they eat.

Reduces Parkinson's risk. According to the National Institutes of Health, drinking one to four cups of green tea a day seems to protect people against developing Parkinson's disease.

Lowers cholesterol. According to the University of Maryland Medical Center's alternative medicine database, green tea lowers total cholesterol and raises HDL (good) cholesterol, and men who drink green tea are more likely to have lower total cholesterol than those who don't drink it.

Potentially protects against cancer. We know that in countries where people drink lots of green tea, cancer rates tend to be lower—and, as a matter of fact, drinking black tea also seems to offer a protective edge against the disease. We know the most about green tea's breast cancer benefits: In one study of 472 women with breast cancer in various stages, the women who drank the most green tea had the least spread of cancer. The effect was greatest for postmenopausal women in the earliest stages of cancer. The researchers also learned that women in the early stages of breast cancer who drank at least five cups of tea a day before their diagnosis were less likely to have recurrences of the disease after they finished treatment.

What about Herbal Teas?

Teas made from medicinal herbs are wonderfully helpful for many of the conditions you might be dealing with or trying to avoid. In my experience, drinking medicinal tea can sometimes replace taking pills, under the right circumstances. You'll find specific recommendations for herbal teas in the conditions chapters in Part II.

Unfortunately, drinking green tea didn't help women with late-stage breast cancer. And finally, in one very large study, women under the age of 50 who drank three or more cups of green tea a day were 37 percent less likely to develop breast cancer compared with women who weren't green tea drinkers.

Could help balance blood sugar. In traditional medicine, healers use green tea to help control blood sugar levels; drinking green tea may be helpful in stabilizing blood sugar. And a number of Chinese studies have shown that drinking green tea decreases fasting glucose and lowers A1C numbers, which is why I make sure that my patients who have diabetes drink green tea regularly.[44, 45]

Black Tea

Like its green cousin, black tea is made from the leaves of the *Camellia sinensis* plant. But green tea is brewed from fresh tea leaves; black tea leaves are aged. In addition to its 2 to 4 percent caffeine content, black tea also contains antioxidants and other compounds that appear to protect the heart and blood vessels. Among black tea's benefits are:

Improved alertness. Like any other beverage containing caffeine, black tea helps keep you alert and sharp.

Reduced stroke risk. Researchers who investigated the relationship between stroke and green or black tea drinking discovered that people who drank more than three cups of either tea a day lowered their risk for stroke by 21 percent.[46]

Reduced heart attack risk. Not only can drinking black tea reduce your heart attack risk, but your heart attack is less likely to be a fatal one if you've been drinking black tea for more than 1 year.

Slightly reduced kidney stone risk. Studies show that women who drink black tea have an 8 percent lower risk of developing kidney stones.

Reduced ovarian cancer risk. Women who are regular tea drinkers— both green and black—have a significantly lower risk for developing ovarian cancer compared with women who rarely or never drink tea.[47]

Which Tea Is Best?

You have a nearly overwhelming number of options when it comes to choosing a tea. Supermarket shelves offer a multitude of different boxes of tea bags from which you can brew a cup or pitcher of green or black tea. You'll also find an increasingly wide array of bottled teas. Which is best—bottled or brewed? And here's another question you might be asking yourself: Does hot tea have any advantages over iced tea?

When *Prevention* magazine recently conducted its own study of this topic, the editors delivered a few surprise findings. After sending samples off to a lab to analyze the teas' antioxidant content, here's what they learned when comparing options.

Homemade iced tea vs. bottled tea. Winner: Homemade (made by brewing tea bags in hot water, then chilling) had more antioxidants than bottled teas. However, two commercial teas also delivered spectacular antioxidant power: Honest Tea Moroccan Mint (bottled green tea) and Lipton's Cold Brew tea bags, which even outscored blueberries, the fruit that's highest in antioxidant power.

Hot brewed vs. fridge brewed. Winner: Believe it or not, fridge-brewed tea beat out hot-brewed iced tea made from the same box of Salada tea bags. The answer might be agitation: The fridge tea might have been stirred or agitated more than the hot-brewed tea; agitation ups antioxidant release.

Green tea vs. black. Winner: A tie. Both green and black teas delivered high antioxidant levels. Which should you drink? We vote for drinking several cups a day of both kinds of tea for maximum antipill power.[48]

No matter which type of tea you choose, please make it organic, and be sure the tea bags are made from unbleached paper.

Coffee

You may not think of coffee as a health drink, but the research that's been consistently piling up in its favor should convince you otherwise. First, here's a fact that may have escaped your attention: Coffee turns out to be the number one source of antioxidants in the American diet, say researchers at the University of Scranton in Pennsylvania. Sipping just a cup or two a day is enough to deliver coffee's load of pill-kicking antioxidant benefits. Plus, decaf is as antioxidant-rich as caffeinated coffee. When it comes to decaf, however, read the labels and buy only water-processed decaf. Most commercially decaffeinated coffee is made using a process that employs potentially harmful chemicals.

Studies on coffee have turned up promising evidence for some key health benefits.

Protects against heart disease. Researchers at Beth Israel Deaconess

Medical Center in Boston and Harvard School of Public Health concluded that drinking coffee in moderation protects against heart failure. In their study, "moderation" equaled two 8-ounce servings of coffee a day.

Lowers the risk of type 2 diabetes. Researchers investigating cancer and nutrition in a huge (43,659 participants) 2012 European study discovered, after nearly 9 years of follow-up, that coffee drinkers (decaf or regular) had a lower risk for type 2 diabetes than did those who did not drink coffee.[49]

Additionally, researchers studying 3,837 Finnish patients with type 2 diabetes in 2006 discovered that the more coffee a patient drank, the lower his risk of dying from heart disease.[50]

Decreases risk of Parkinson's disease. Researchers in an early 2000 study linked coffee drinking with a significantly lower risk for developing Parkinson's disease.

Reduces liver problems. Your favorite eye-opener also seems to be particularly liver-friendly. Italian researchers showed that drinking coffee can lower liver cancer risk by about 40 percent; drinking three cups a day slashes risk to about 50 percent. And a study from Kaiser Permanente in Oakland, California, points to coffee's ability to lower the incidence of liver cirrhosis in alcohol drinkers by 22 percent. Finally, a 2014 study published in the journal *Hepatology* suggests that drinking two or more cups of coffee daily reduces the risk of death from liver cirrhosis by 66 percent.[51]

What Not to Drink: "Diet" Drinks

Sugary sodas and overly sweetened fruity drinks aren't included in the No More Pills Plan. An overwhelming chorus of health experts points to sugary drinks as at least partially to blame for our obesity and diabetes crises. So I won't reiterate all the reasons why you won't be drinking sweetened soft drinks on this plan—and why you shouldn't drink them, period, even when you're *off* the plan.

But artificial sweeteners are also squarely off the plan. I do think it's important to let you know how devious these sweeteners are, on the chance that you're not committed to breaking up with your beloved diet drinks quite yet. Take it from me: Please do!

Talk about a historically controversial product—fake sweeteners have stirred up concerns ever since they came to market in the 1800s. First, researchers worried that these sweeteners could cause cancer, which, decades later, seemed to become a self-fulfilling prophecy. Headlines went national in the 1960s when the FDA first banned cyclamates and then saccharin due to research findings that they caused cancer in lab animals. Later, we learned that the poor lab rats in those studies were fed more artificial sweeteners than a normal human could possibly encounter in real life—and that, said the researchers, did not translate to a cancer risk in humans. The ban on saccharin was later lifted.[52]

Then along came aspartame, another artificial sweetener made from the naturally occurring amino acids aspartic acid and phenylalanine. It ran into trouble when users complained about experiencing headaches, depression, increased hunger, and even incidences of cancer.

It turns out that studies on aspartame weren't as clear as we might wish. But one medical authority, neurologist Russell Blaylock, MD, has written extensively about harm to the brain from aspartame (and MSG) in his excellent book, *Excitotoxins: The Taste That Kills*. I follow his recommendations and make sure that all of my patients avoid both of these items. After all, I've seen it for myself: Many of my patients react badly to aspartame. I tell all of my patients to absolutely avoid any artificially sweetened beverage (or food). And one group of people must be extremely careful to avoid the fake stuff: People who have the rare genetic metabolism disorder phenylketonuria (PKU) can't break down phenylalanine, which causes various and potentially serious problems.

If you ask me, the most fascinating aspect of the artificial sugar controversy is that researchers have started implicating fake sugar in America's obesity epidemic. Talk about unintended consequences! After all, artificial sweeteners were invented to help people stop drinking sugar-sweetened beverages and to make their weight loss and antidiabetes efforts easier to accomplish. But researchers have come up with the following startling revelations:

- A 2009 study published in *Diabetes Care* suggests that drinking diet sodas every day could increase your risk of type 2 diabetes by 67 percent.

- A 2011 study published in the *American Journal of Clinical Nutrition* points to the fact that diet soft drinks increase fat storage in the liver.

- A study presented at the 2011 American Diabetes Association's Scientific Sessions pointed to the possibility that drinking diet sodas could expand your waistline.

However, a research study arrived in the fall of 2014 that literally took my breath away. Conducted in Israel at several leading medical and research facilities, the study looked at the way sweeteners affect beneficial gut bacteria in both lab animals and humans. Here's what the researchers learned: Artificial sweeteners actually alter gut bacteria in a way that triggers glucose intolerance. That's huge, people.

In their study, the researchers made a remarkable (and in my opinion, shocking) statement: "Artificial sweeteners were extensively introduced into our diets with the intention of reducing caloric intake and normalizing blood glucose levels without compromising the human 'sweet tooth.' This increase in non-caloric artificial sweeteners coincides with the dramatic increase in the obesity and diabetes epidemics." The researchers connected the dots between the sweeteners and the epidemics, and said, "Artificial sweeteners may have directly contributed to enhancing the epidemic they were intended to fight."[53]

I agree. Unsweetened is the way to go when it comes to your beverages. At most, ½ teaspoon of organic honey, maple syrup, or agave nectar should provide all the sweetness you need. Just don't overdo it.

A (Happy) Word on Wine

And where does the No More Pills Plan stand on your nightly glass of wine? The press can be confusing. You might hear that a drink or two is good for your heart, that it can lessen the risk for type 2 diabetes, or that it can even protect you against Alzheimer's disease. Or you'll hear that drinking raises the risks for those very diseases and that you're at higher risk for breast cancer if you're a woman who drinks. Where's the truth?[54, 55]

It's all about moderation—and moderation, for most people, is much less alcohol than you'd think: just two drinks a day for men and only one for women. In the good-for-you column, one nightly glass of wine can raise levels of good HDL cholesterol. It can lower blood pressure, prevent artery damage caused by bad LDL cholesterol, and reduce your risk for blood clots, says the American Heart Association. I recommend that if my patients want to drink wine, they limit it to one small glass of organic, nonsulfited wine with dinner, and not every day—generally four or five times a week at most.

But for some people—such as those who have heart failure, high blood pressure, diabetes, or, for that matter, any chronic illness—drinking even one glass a night is something to discuss with your doctor, especially if you're taking any medications.[56]

Your Weekly Sample Meal Plan

The best thing about the No More Pills Plan is how delectable the food is and how satisfied you'll feel from eating this way. Though I haven't designed this as a weight loss diet (unless you're thinking about the weight of all those pills you'll be losing!), chances are, if you're overweight, you'll probably shed several pounds (or more) without even trying, because you won't be eating fast or junk food or sugary desserts on this plan.

Here's what a week's worth of meals might look like; just follow the do's and don'ts in this chapter and you can easily create yummy dishes like these.

MONDAY

Breakfast: 3-egg omelet with chopped bell peppers and onions
Snack: Nut and Seed Clusters (page 301)
Lunch: Fish and Chips (page 269)
Dinner: Roast beef salad or stir-fry with veggies and mushrooms

Snack: Roasted Kale Chips (page 295)
   or . . .
Dessert: Peach Melba (page 303)

TUESDAY

Breakfast: Super Strawberry Smoothie (page 261)
Snack: Baked Apple (page 292)
Lunch: Noodle Bowl (page 263)
Dinner: Tuna, avocado, and broccoli lettuce wrap

Snack: Spiced Pecans (page 293)
   or . . .
Dessert: Crustless Apple Crumb Pie (page 302)

WEDNESDAY

Breakfast: 3-egg omelet with chopped bell peppers and onions
Snack: Avocado Salsa with carrot and celery sticks (page 300)
Lunch: Hearty Vegetable Soup (page 265)
Dinner: Szechuan Chicken (page 289)

Snack: Roasted Kale Chips (page 295)
  or . . .
Dessert: Frothy Hot Chocolate (page 290)

THURSDAY

Breakfast: Poached eggs on spinach
Snack: Roasted Kale Chips (page 295)
Lunch: Pan-Seared Fish Tacos (page 271)
Dinner: Shepherd's Pie (page 276)

Snack: 5 celery sticks stuffed with almond or cashew butter
  or . . .
Dessert: Strawberry or Peach Coconut Milk Ice Cream (page 299)

FRIDAY

Breakfast: Chocolate-Almond Smoothie (page 298)
Snack: Snackin' Nuts (page 294)
Lunch: Salmon-Avocado Wraps (page 264)
Dinner: Pistachio-Crusted Chicken Breast (page 283)

Snack: Eggplant Dip with raw veggies (page 304)
  or . . .
Dessert: Marinated Summer Berries (page 291)

SATURDAY

Breakfast: Scrambled eggs with mushrooms
Snack: Frothy Hot Chocolate (page 290)
Lunch: Roasted Chicken and Spinach Salad (page 266)
Dinner: Tuscan Tuna Cakes (page 279)

Snack: Nut and Seed Clusters (page 301)
  or . . .
Dessert: Crustless Apple Crumb Pie (page 302)

SUNDAY

Breakfast: Poached eggs on spinach

Snack: Baked Pumpkin Pudding (page 297)

Lunch: Tangy Roast Beef Lettuce Wraps (page 270)

Dinner: Spaghetti Squash Casserole (page 288)

Snack: Eggplant Dip and raw veggies (page 304)
or . . .
Dessert: Peach Melba (page 303)

Final Considerations

I've done a lot of myth busting here and presented you with a set of guidelines that go "against the grain" (pun intended) of years of diet recommendations. As Americans, we're used to the low-fat diet, the food pyramid, the milk mustache campaigns, the food industry and its insidious use of mouthfeel (combining trans fats and other health-killing ingredients that feel comforting when we eat them) and its addictive strategies that make us crave unhealthy foods.

My response is to ask, so how's that working for us? Why are we dealing with a national obesity epidemic? Why are there so many kids with middle-aged shapes and middle-aged diseases? Bottom line: Eating what the food industry wants you to eat is like surfing a deadly fast lane. At its end, you'll slam into the cascade of chronic diseases that await people who follow the terribly unhealthy, so-called Western diet. And with that comes a medicine chest full of pills and those plastic boxes sectioned off so that you know which pills to take all day long.

Chapter 4

Downsize Your Pills with Activity

The perfect exercise program is like a three-legged chair—you need all three legs to hold yourself up. When it comes to exercise, that means three components: aerobics, muscle strengthening, and stretching. The No More Pills Plan fulfills all three components with an aerobic walking plan, an easy strength-training program, and a relaxing yoga routine that helps keep you flexible.

This is a plan for life that, unlike so many other exercise programs, is not specifically designed to help you lose weight or burn calories (those realities will, however, be your happy by-products of following the plan). You'll feel immediately better just a week or two after starting the program—so good, in fact, that I bet you'll want to stick with it forever. That would be a good thing, because study after study shows that being consistently active over time is the key to warding off chronic diseases—and keeping those pill bottles at bay.

The Sitting Disease

Here's one disease your doctor won't prescribe pills for—in fact, she may not even diagnose it. But she absolutely should, because sitting is actually killing us; it's almost as deadly over time as some of our most serious chronic

We Can Do Better

When it comes to fitness, sadly, most of us are in pretty underwhelming shape. In fact, according to the latest (2011) statistics from the Centers for Disease Control and Prevention, 52 percent of American adults didn't meet nationally recognized recommendations for aerobic exercise or physical activity. And 76 percent of us didn't meet recommendations for doing muscle-strengthening activities.[1]

diseases. And despite the fact that studies show that exercise is as effective as pills for heart disease, for example, only one-third of primary care doctors even mention it, much less prescribe it.

Here's the scary truth: A couch potato lifestyle increases your risks for chronic disease. In fact, inactivity is so unhealthy that it's actually called the *sitting disease*. For example, a couple of years ago, researchers did some digging into the television-watching habits of Australians. They learned something pretty horrifying: The amount of TV people viewed in Australia in 2008 reduced life expectancy by *nearly 2 years for men and 1.5 years for women*. They also discovered that people who watched the most TV shortened their lives even more—6 hours a day for a lifetime of boob-tube watching translated to a lifetime nearly 5 years shorter than that of folks who didn't watch TV. Another grim statistic: *Every single hour of TV you watch after the age of 25 reduces your life expectancy by nearly 22 minutes.*[2]

It might be time to post this sign on top of your TV: "Is watching another *Law & Order* rerun really worth shaving 22 minutes off my life?"

It's not the brain-numbing aspects of television watching that shorten your life—it's the inactivity. We know for a fact that inactivity contributes to disease. Here are just a few of inactivity's insidious effects.

- The less active you are, the higher your risk for developing high blood pressure.

- Inactive people are more likely to develop heart disease than active people are.

- Inactivity may increase your risk for certain cancers.
- If you're active, even if you're overweight or obese, your risk for disease drops significantly.
- Lack of activity contributes to depression and anxiety.[3]

So what happens once you become active? You start fending off diseases instead of developing them. As an example, in 2007, researchers combed through studies that linked exercise with decreased risk of chronic disease and discovered that people who exercised regularly reaped some pretty sweet benefits. They dropped their risks for breast cancer by 75 percent, for heart disease by 49 percent, for diabetes by 35 percent, and for colorectal cancer by 22 percent.[4]

It doesn't even take as much activity as you might think to turn things around. In fact, *overdoing* exercise is as unhealthy as being inactive. In their 2014 *Heart* study that examined exercise and its benefits for people with heart disease, German researchers revealed a bit of a surprise. As you'd expect, people with heart disease who rarely or never exercise have a much worse prognosis than people who engage in strenuous activity (defined as "sweat-inducing activities such as cycling, speedy hiking, gardening, or a sport") two to four times a week. What surprised the researchers, however, was this: They learned that people who performed strenuous exercise five to six times a week had the same number of major cardiovascular events as did people who rarely or never exercised.[5]

The results of that study confirm what I've been telling my patients. I want them to be active three to four times a week, for a total weekly minimum of 90 minutes to a maximum of 160 minutes.

Walking Is Your Best Medicine

It's unlikely that you remember that earthshaking day when you took your very first steps. But whoever was lucky enough to be watching you probably would, and it's likely that your audience burst into cheers of joy back then when you first put one tiny foot in front of the other and teetered across the floor. Too bad you don't hear cheers of joy every time you go walking as an adult—maybe if you did, it would be motivation enough for you to do some walking every day!

Walking is among the best things you can do to prevent the kinds of illnesses that prompt your doctor to prescribe pills. Let's take a look at the science; it offers a number of pretty compelling reasons to make walking a part of your life. Here's what walking can do for you.

Lower cholesterol. In their 2014 study, Chinese researchers assigned 330 people with high cholesterol to one of three groups. One group did nothing; the other two groups walked for 30 minutes at least 5 days a week. One group walked in the morning; the other group walked in the evening. The researchers measured all participants' cholesterol and checked them for signs of system-wide inflammation at the start and finish of the 12-week study. The result? Walking lowered participants' cholesterol in both groups, and it also lowered their inflammation markers. Interestingly, the evening walkers posted better results than did the morning walkers.[6] So the bottom line here is that walking puts you on a path to lowering or maybe even stopping your cholesterol drugs. What's more, when you lower your markers for body-wide inflammation, you also lower your chances of developing inflammation-driven diseases such as heart disease, diabetes, and arthritis, to name just a few.

Improve metabolic syndrome. In 2013, Italian researchers studied the effects of a walking program on 176 people with metabolic syndrome—a diagnosis that includes borderline high cholesterol, blood glucose, and waist circumference measurements. Participants were asked to walk at a brisk pace for an hour a day, 5 days a week, for 24 weeks. When participants were tested at the end of the study, their A1C levels (a marker for blood glucose over time) had dropped, their good cholesterol levels had risen, and their total cholesterol and triglyceride levels also had dropped. They also lost about 2 inches off their waist circumference.[7]

Help prevent heart attacks and strokes. In a study of 72,488 nurses, those who walked at least 3 hours a week had a 35 percent lower risk of heart attacks and cardiac death and a 34 percent lower risk of stroke. In another study of 44,452 male health professionals, walking at least 30 minutes a day lowered their risk for coronary artery disease by 18 percent.[8]

Help keep you alive. Now there's a great reason to walk, right? Researchers who looked at the health records of 10,269 male graduates of Harvard College reported that those who walked at least 9 miles a week had a 22 percent lower death rate than did nonwalkers.[9]

Why I Love Interval Walking

I encourage my patients to walk 30 to 40 minutes a day, at least three to four times a week. It doesn't matter if you walk outdoors (which is wonderful if you have a safe, scenic route available and the weather isn't treacherous) or indoors on a track, a treadmill, or an elliptical machine. For that matter, if you prefer, you can also ride a bike or a stationary exercise bike.

If you haven't been active for months or years, please start slowly and go at a pace that feels comfortable for you. Personally, I like to start my day with a walk, and if the weather isn't welcoming, then I just hop on my stationary bike.

I like to add interval work to my walks. This means that you walk at your absolute fastest pace for 20 to 30 seconds or so. Then you slow down and walk at a slow to normal pace for 2 minutes as your heart rate goes down. Then you speed it up again for another 20 to 30 seconds. Repeat for a total of three times. You can also do your intervals on a stationary bike, a treadmill, an elliptical machine—you get the idea. The goal is to work at your maximum capacity for a very short time, recover, and then repeat. Once you've done this for a while, you'll find that you're probably able to go a little faster and stretch it out a little longer during your speed intervals.

Though it may sound like a silly way to exercise, interval work offers benefits that will help you succeed in your quest to lower or stop taking your pills. And I like the fact that during your workout, you're actually only really pushing yourself for a minute or so, while you're more or less cruising for the rest of the time. Doing intervals seems to make my exercise time fly by.

What's more, there's one incredibly important reason why interval work is an important feature of the No More Pills Plan, and that's the way it helps melt "belly fat."[10] You may think of your tummy simply as excess flab that makes your jeans hard to button, but belly fat is far more insidious than a simple cosmetic problem.

Unlike fat deposits on your thighs, butt, or upper arms, the belly fat that lies deep within your abdomen actually acts in a very similar way to an organ—an evil organ. Unlike the "good" organs—your stomach, intestines, and liver, for example—that keep you alive, the fat that surrounds them produces toxic, inflammatory compounds. When your internal fat secretes these chemicals, it sparks cascades of intricate interactions that (among many other damaging effects) weaken your heart, damage your blood vessels, and dampen your immunity.

If you have diabetes, having excess belly fat is an even bigger danger because it makes your body less sensitive to insulin. It increases insulin resistance, meaning that it takes more and more insulin to take glucose into the cells. Carrying too much fat around your middle puts you on the fast track to beta-cell failure. These are the cells in the pancreas that produce insulin; when they burn out completely or partially, you end up taking drugs for the rest of your life. And you'll also be more likely to experience diabetic complications, including heart problems, kidney failure, cognitive difficulties, vision problems, and problems with your feet.[11] Bottom line: Whittling away as much belly fat as you can is a key to success when you're trying to say no to pills. And doing interval work is a great way to accomplish that.

The No More Pills Walking Program

The No More Pills Walking Program is structured to get you up and moving regularly. Its beauty is that it gently eases you into an activity routine, so it's excellent for people who've been sedentary for a while. If walking for 15 minutes at first is too much for you, no worries. Just start with a 5-minute or 10-minute walk and progress from there. These strategies can help you turn into a person who walks regularly—and loves it.

Find your path. Pick a place to walk that's both visually appealing and convenient. This might mean the fresh air and nature you'll find at a nearby park or walking path. Or you may prefer heading to your local gym and using a treadmill or elliptical machine. For some, it's the local mall—just stash your wallet, and whatever you do, avoid the food court!

Walk proud. Walking with poor posture or technique can leave you vulnerable to unnecessary pain or injuries. Make sure you're standing straight with your shoulders down and chin parallel to the ground. Tuck in your tummy and bend your arms at a 90-degree angle. Make sure the heel of your foot meets the ground first before your foot rolls forward, and push off from your toes. Tip: Walk lightly with a spring in your step, and wear good shoes. Too heavy a heel-strike or bad shoes can bring on heel pain and plantar fasciitis.

Find a pal. Sometimes a walking friend can provide the extra support you need to maintain your walking program. Consider asking your spouse, coworker, or neighbor to join you on your walks. Studies have shown that those new to fitness plans are more likely to stick to their routines if they have a partner.

Make it fun. Whether you're starting off with a walk of 5 minutes or 15 minutes, it's important to challenge yourself during each walk. Try to increase your pace or your time, or both—but don't push yourself so hard that you risk an injury. Something as simple as listening to music can make your walks more enjoyable. You can change the song when you change your intensity level to aid in increasing or decreasing your pace. Or you might find it fun to try one of the fitness trackers that monitor your distance and heart rate and provide motivation.

Giving Some Thought to Your Walking Program

Take a few moments to think about the other benefits you may want to get from your walking regimen. While this program is designed to help you ward off illness and hopefully lessen your dependence on prescription medication, you can also use your walking time to mentally sort through your daily to-do list, listen to some soothing music, or even just take a break and clear your mind.

So, in the space below, jot down some beneficial ways you can make the most out of your 15-minute walk.

_____

_____

_____

_____

_____

_____

_____

THE 2-WEEK NO MORE PILLS WALKING PLAN

As you progress, be sure to add 30-second intervals into the moderate-pace phase.

WEEK 1		
Day 1	**Total Workout Time**	**The Routine**
	15 minutes	5 minutes (easy pace) 5 minutes (moderate pace) 5 minutes (easy pace)
Day 2	REST	
Day 3	**Total Workout Time**	**The Routine**
	15 minutes	4 minutes (easy pace) 7 minutes (moderate pace) 4 minutes (easy pace)
Day 4	**Total Workout Time**	**The Routine**
	20 minutes	5 minutes (easy pace) 10 minutes (moderate pace) 5 minutes (easy pace)
Day 5	REST	
Day 6	**Total Workout Time**	**The Routine**
	15 minutes	3 minutes (easy pace) 9 minutes (moderate pace) 3 minutes (easy pace)
Day 7	REST	

WEEK 2		
	Total Workout Time	**The Routine**
Day **8**	20 minutes	5 minutes (easy pace) 10 minutes (moderate pace) 5 minutes (easy pace)
Day **9**	REST	
	Total Workout Time	**The Routine**
Day **10**	15 minutes	2 minutes (easy pace) 10 minutes (moderate pace) 3 minutes (easy pace)
	Total Workout Time	**The Routine**
Day **11**	25 minutes	5 minutes (easy pace) 15 minutes (moderate pace) 5 minutes (easy pace)
	Total Workout Time	**The Routine**
Day **12**	20 minutes	4 minutes (easy pace) 12 minutes (moderate pace) 4 minutes (easy pace)
	Total Workout Time	**The Routine**
Day **13**	30 minutes	5 minutes (easy pace) 20 minutes (moderate pace) 5 minutes (easy pace)
Day **14**	REST	

After you've completed the 2-week plan, you can maintain it by repeating the routine for Day 13, making sure to add at least five 1-minute intervals of "fast as you can" walking during the moderate 20-minute phase of the walk. And make sure you allow your heart to slow back down to normal before you do another interval.

Get Stronger, Live Longer, Take Fewer Pills

Keeping muscles strong is a key to beating the frailty that can accompany aging. The truth is that as we get older, it's really all about "use it or lose it." That's because unless you work your muscles, your overall strength will decline significantly after age 50—at the rate of something like 15 percent per decade. That's why I want you to include a gentle weight-training program, using light weights, and I want you to work at a very comfortable pace. Over time, you can increase the weight and repetitions as your muscles get stronger. All it takes is 15 minutes per session 2 days a week.

Trust me, you won't end up looking like a muscle-bound weight lifter. But doing these muscle-strengthening exercises regularly will increase your muscle strength, improve your metabolism and bone density, decrease your insulin resistance, and help you sleep better. Don't neglect exercises for your core muscles, those that support your lower back and abdomen. Working these muscles helps improve your balance and stability, lessening your risk of falls.

Just Starting Out? Over 55? Begin with These.

Do 8 to 10 repetitions of each exercise for 2 sets. After 4 weeks, you should be able to move on to the No More Pills 4-Week Strength-Training Program.

For all strength-training exercises:

- Complete all movements in a slow, controlled fashion.
- Don't hold your breath.
- Stop if you feel pain.
- Stretch each muscle after your workout.

Wall Pushups: Place your hands flat against a wall. Slowly lower your body to the wall. Push your body away from the wall to return to the starting position.

Chair Squats: Begin by sitting in a chair. Lean slightly forward and stand up from the chair. Try not to favor one side or use your hands to help you.

Biceps Curls: Hold a weight in each hand with your arms at your sides. Bending your arms at the elbows, lift the weights to your shoulders and then lower them to your sides.

Shoulder Shrugs: Hold a weight in each hand with your arms at your sides. Shrug your shoulders up toward your ears and then lower them back down.[12]

The No More Pills
4-Week Strength-Training Program

Try this 2-day-a-week program first if you're under age 55 and already conditioned. If you are older and have spent 4 weeks regularly performing the beginner exercises and are ready for more of a challenge, you can also give this program a try—though you might want to use the "Make It Easier" moves for the first week or so. Use 2-pound weights at first, and then graduate to 3-pound weights after the first 2 weeks.

Once you've completed the 4-week program, you can add a set of reps as well as a fourth workout each week. When your 3-pound weights become very easy to lift, use 5-pound weights. Be sure to rest 1 day between your workout sessions.

THE 4-WEEK STRENGTH-TRAINING PROGRAM

WEEK	DAY 1	DAY 2	DAY 3 (optional)	DAY 4	DAY 5	DAY 6	DAY 7
1	OFF	2 sets, 10 reps, 45–60 seconds rest	OFF	OFF	2 sets, 10 reps, 45–60 seconds rest	OFF	OFF
2	OFF	2 sets, 12 reps, 30–45 seconds rest	OFF	OFF	2 sets, 12 reps, 30–45 seconds rest	OFF	OFF
3	2 sets, 15 reps, 45–60 seconds rest	OFF	2 sets, 12 reps, 30–45 seconds rest	OFF	2 sets, 10 reps, 15–30 seconds rest	OFF	OFF
4	2 sets, 15 reps, 45–60 seconds rest	OFF	2 sets, 12 reps, 30–45 seconds rest	OFF	2 sets, 10 reps, 15–30 seconds rest	OFF	OFF

The Exercises

1. Squat Sweep
(works the quadriceps, hamstrings, inner thighs, and glutes)

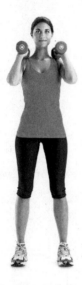

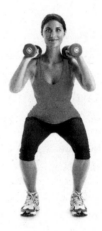

Start Position: Stand with your feet shoulder-width apart, holding a dumbbell in each hand. Curl the weights up until the ends rest on the front of your shoulders.

A. Keeping your back straight, slowly bend your hips and sit back into a half squat.

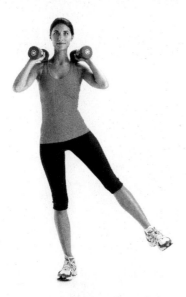

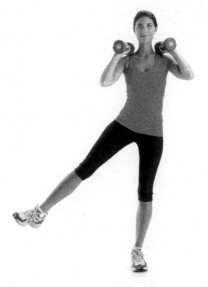

B. As you stand back up, lift your left leg straight out to your side as if you were going to step out. Shoot for raising your foot about 3 inches off the floor, but avoid raising your leg any higher than hip height. Pause for 1 second, then return your foot to the floor so you're back in the start position.

C. Repeat the exercise, this time lifting your right leg out to the side.

D. Alternate legs between every squat for the entire set.

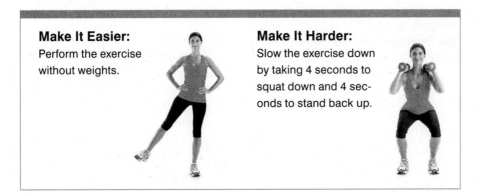

Make It Easier:
Perform the exercise without weights.

Make It Harder:
Slow the exercise down by taking 4 seconds to squat down and 4 seconds to stand back up.

2. Double Chest Press + Fly
(works the chest, shoulders, and triceps)

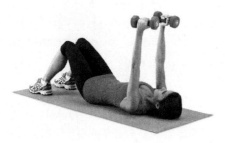

Start Position: Lie faceup on the floor (or a bench), holding a light dumbbell in each hand, knees bent, feet flat on the floor. Raise your arms straight above your chest with your palms facing each other.

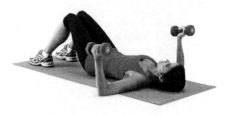

A. Bend your elbows out to your sides and slowly lower the weights until your upper arms touch the floor. (Your palms should stay facing each other as you go.)

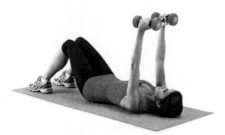

B. Press the weights back up into the start position, then repeat the move once more. This is the chest press.

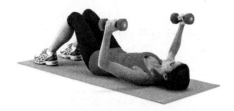

C. Next, slowly sweep your arms out to your sides and down as far as you can. Reverse the motion by sweeping your arms back up in front of you (as if you're hugging someone) until they're back in the start position. This is the fly. Alternate between 2 presses and 1 fly for the recommended amount of repetitions.

Make It Easier:

Once your upper arms touch the floor, rest for 1 second before pushing the weights back into the start position.

Make It Harder:

Lie on a stability ball with your head, shoulders, and upper back supported by the ball; your knees should be bent and your feet flat on the floor. Your body should be one straight line from your head to your knees.

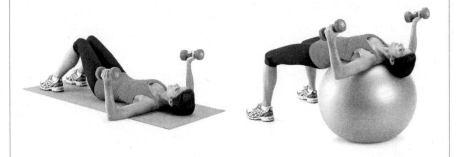

3. Lunge

(works the quadriceps, hamstrings, and glutes)

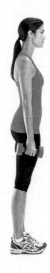 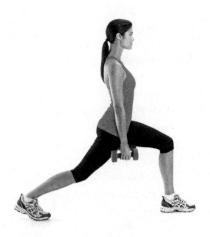

Start Position: Stand straight with a dumbbell in each hand, your arms hanging straight down from your sides, and your palms facing in.

A. Take a big step forward with your left foot and lower your body until your left thigh is almost parallel to the floor. (Your right leg should be extended behind you with only the ball of your right foot on the floor.)

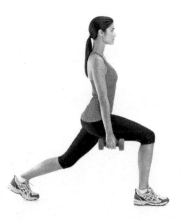

B. Reverse the motion by pressing yourself back into the start position, then repeat the exercise by stepping forward with your right foot. Alternate between stepping forward with your left and right feet throughout the set.

Make It Easier:

Do the exercise without any weights (hands on hips), or try a reverse lunge instead. Stand with your feet together, then step back about 2 to 3 feet with your right foot. Bend your left knee and slowly lower yourself down. (Your left knee should stay directly over your ankle.) Stop right before your right knee touches the floor, then push off with your right foot to get back into the start position. Repeat the move with your left leg.

Make It Harder:

Try turning the movement into a traveling lunge. Instead of stepping back into the start position, keep your front foot planted, then bring the leg that's behind you forward and raise your knee up in front of you. (You'll be balancing on just your front leg.) Plant your foot back down so your feet are even once more.

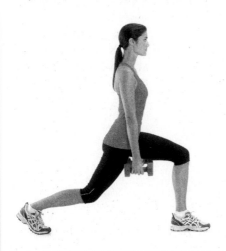
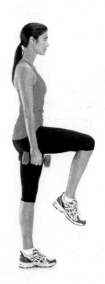

4. Unilateral Bent-Over Row
(works the latissimus dorsi, rhomboids, lower back, and core)

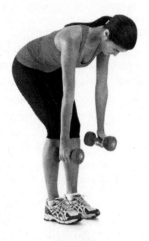
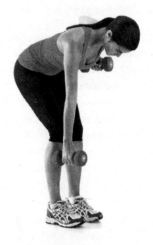

Start Position: Stand with your feet shoulder-width apart, holding a light dumbbell in each hand with an overhand grip, knees slightly bent. Bend forward at your hips until your torso is almost parallel to the floor. Your arms should be hanging straight beneath you, palms facing each other.

A. Keeping your elbows close to your body, pull the weight in your left hand up to the side of your chest. (Your right arm will stay straight.)

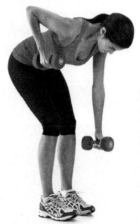

B. Lower the weight in your left hand back down as you simultaneously pull the weight in your right hand up to your side. Continue alternating back and forth for the entire set.

Make It Easier:

Try doing the exercise one arm at a time. To support your lower back, place one hand on a sturdy chair, then bend forward until your torso is at a 45-degree angle to the floor. Do the required repetitions for one arm, then switch positions to work your other arm.

Make It Harder:

Every 1 or 2 repetitions, pull both weights up along your sides, then push your heels into the floor and straighten back up into a standing position, keeping the weights locked into your sides as you go. Immediately reverse the motion, bending forward at the waist first, then lower the weights back down by straightening your arms.

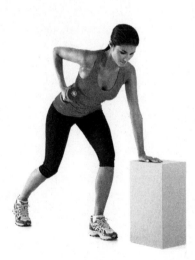

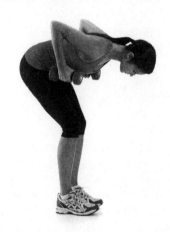

5. Deadlift Curl Press

(works the trapezius, lower back, glutes, hamstrings, shoulders, triceps, and biceps)

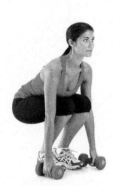 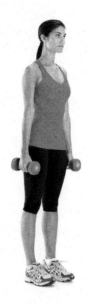 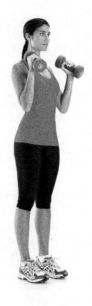

Start Position: Stand with your feet 6 to 8 inches apart with a dumbbell placed along the outside of each foot. Bend your knees and grab the dumbbells so that your palms face in toward each other. Before you begin the exercise, make sure that your back and shoulders are straight (not rounded) and your head is up.

A. With head and back straight, slowly stand up until your legs are straight, knees unlocked, keeping the dumbbells close to your body as you lift.

B. Without moving your upper arms, bend your elbows and curl the weights up to the front of your shoulders, palms facing each other.

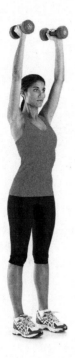

C. Press the weights up over your head until your arms are straight, elbows unlocked, palms facing each other. Reverse the entire exercise until you're back in the start position.

Make It Easier:

Instead of starting the exercise with the weights on the floor, place them on a pair of sturdy boxes. This will prevent you from having to lower yourself down as far, which makes the move much simpler to perform.

Make It Harder:

Try pausing a few times during the exercise. This will keep your muscles under a longer duration of tension so you utilize even more muscle fibers. During each repetition:

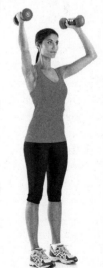

• Pause for 1 second during the deadlift portion (when your thighs are at a 45-degree angle as you rise up).
• Pause for 1 second during the curl portion (when your forearms are parallel to the floor).
• Pause for 1 second during the pressing portion (when your arms are bent at 90-degree angles).

6. Bicycle Crunch
(works the abdominal muscles)

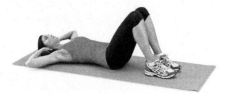 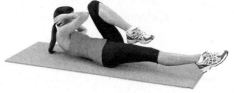

Start Position: Lie faceup on the floor with your knees bent and your feet flat on the floor. Lightly cup your hands over your ears, letting your elbows point out to the sides.

A. Draw your left knee toward your chest while extending your right leg. Simultaneously curl your torso up and twist to the left so that your right elbow and left knee touch (or at least come close to touching).

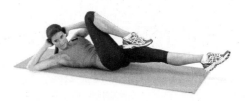

B. Repeat the exercise, this time pulling your right knee in as you curl and twist your torso to the right, touching your left elbow to your right knee. Alternate back and forth from side to side for the entire exercise, keeping your feet off the floor the entire time.

Make It Easier:

Keep your knees bent and your feet on the floor, then raise only one knee at a time, leaving the opposite foot on the floor.

Make It Harder:

Try pausing for 1 or 2 seconds each time your elbow meets your knee. Or better yet, pulse by doing 1 or 2 mini-reps (bringing your knee and elbow together, then apart by an inch or so, then back together again). Either way will keep your abs contracted for a longer period of time.

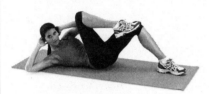

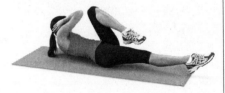

7. Plank
(works the core)

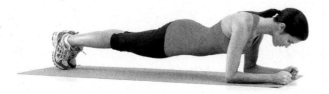

Start Position: Get into a pushup position—legs extended behind you, feet shoulder-width apart, with your weight on your toes. Rest on your forearms so that your arms are at 90-degree angles.

Keeping your head and back straight, hold this position for 30 seconds during Week 1; for each additional week, add between 5 and 10 seconds, depending on your strength level.

Make It Easier:
Bend your legs so that you're resting on one knee (your other leg stays extended) or both knees.

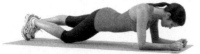

Make It Harder:
Keeping your arms and feet in place, slowly twist and lower your left hip toward the floor. Repeat by twisting the opposite way and lowering your right hip. Alternate back and forth for the entire duration.

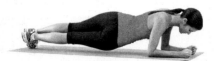

The Easy, Relaxing
No More Pills Yoga Program

Transitioning from being an inactive person to an active person, getting your body fitter, and losing belly fat are three excellent reasons to begin the No More Pills Walking and Strength-Training Programs. Relieving stress, stretching your body, keeping your mind sharp, and improving your balance and coordination are five terrific reasons to add a yoga component. Here are some easy poses that virtually anyone can do.

Note: If you can't hold a pose as long as recommended, ease into Child's Pose and resume when you're ready. The entire routine should take about 30 minutes or so.

Get Started

You'll need a yoga mat; loose, comfortable clothes; and a quiet space. It's good to ease into your yoga practice with a few deep, relaxed breaths.

Pose 1:

Cat-Cow

Start on all fours. Exhale and round your back, tucking your pelvis in (A). Inhale and reverse the motion, arching your back and looking up (B). Do this pose 8 times.

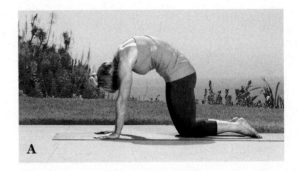

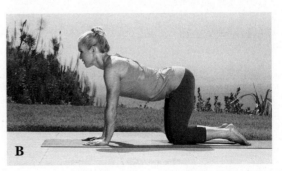

Pose 2:

Arm and Leg Extension

Start on all fours, then exhale and extend your right arm and your left leg. Do 8 times on each side.

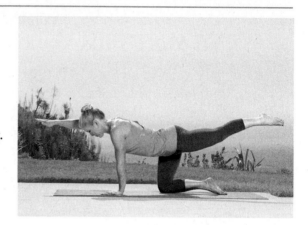

Pose 3:

Child's Pose

Start on all fours, and then sit back on your heels. Lower your forehead to the mat, and reach your arms forward. Hold for 6 to 8 deep breaths.

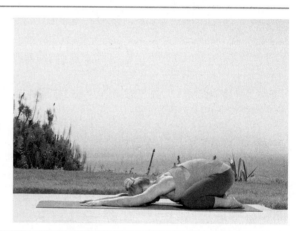

Pose 4:

Downward-Facing Dog

With your palms and toes on the mat, lift your hips to form an upside-down V, pressing your hands and heels into the mat. Relax your head and neck. Hold for 6 to 8 deep breaths.

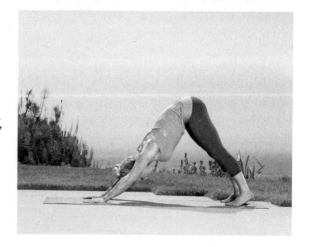

Pose 5:
Plank

With your palms and toes on the mat, lower your hips into a pushup position. Keep your shoulders over your wrists, your abs tight, and your spine long. Hold for 4 deep breaths.

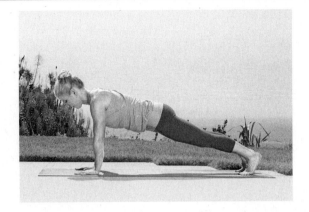

Pose 6:
Hover

From a plank position, bend your elbows, keeping your arms close to your body, and lower your chest almost to the mat. Hold for 4 deep breaths.

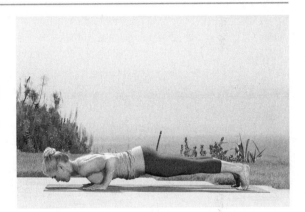

Pose 7:
Cobra

From the hover position, lower your body to the mat. Press into your hands, lift and extend your spine, raise your chest, and look straight ahead. Hold for 4 deep breaths.

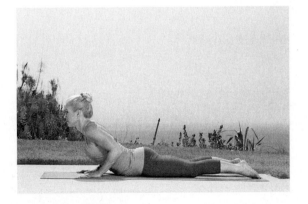

Next

Repeat from Downward-Facing Dog at a slightly faster pace, about 2 breaths per move. Do 4 times, ending in Downward-Facing Dog.

Pose 8:

Warrior 2

Standing up, step your right foot forward into a lunge position, with your right knee bent. Turn your hips to face the side. Extend your arms at shoulder height, palms facing down. Look over your right hand. Hold for 4 to 6 deep breaths.

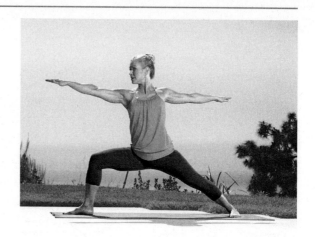

Pose 9:

Reverse Warrior

Lower your left hand to your left leg. Reach your right arm overhead and look up. Hold for 4 to 6 deep breaths.

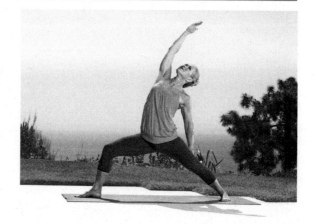

Pose 10:

Side Angle

From a standing position, lower your right forearm to your right thigh. Reach your left arm overhead and look straight up. Hold for 4 to 6 deep breaths.

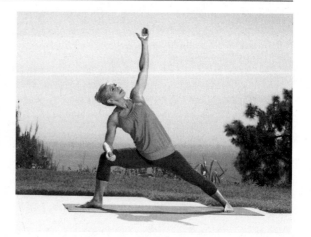

Next

From the Side Angle pose, lower your hands to the mat on either side of your right foot. Step your right foot backward into Downward-Facing Dog. Repeat from Warrior 2 with your left foot forward.

Finish

Starting at Downward-Facing Dog, do the entire sequence 4 times total. Finish in Child's Pose with several deep, calming breaths.

So that's it! Aerobics, strengthening, and stretching—the perfect "triple crown" for your health.

Chapter 5

Coping with Stress

Stress is intricately intertwined with the birth of chronic diseases, so learning to keep your stress levels under control is crucial to the No More Pills Plan. That's because helping you avoid chronic disease, or at least lessening its severity, can also help you lower your medication dosage or perhaps get off your pills altogether. This chapter will explain exactly how stress impacts your health and will outline several simple yet highly effective strategies for taming the insidious influence stress has on your body—and your mind.

But first, let's face it—life without any stress at all would pretty much be a vanilla existence. Stress can be that happy, tingly anticipation you feel when you're waiting for something wonderful to happen—the trip to the airport to embark on your vacation, for example. Who'd want to live without that? On the other hand, stress can also be unpleasantness to the max: think getting stuck in traffic on your way to a job interview. Just picturing that scenario is enough to make your heart start pounding.

We'll never erase those quick-to-pass stressful good and bad moments from our lives, nor would we want to. A bit of stress now and then is the spice we need to stay alert and feel alive. But when stressful moments become chronic, stress becomes dangerous. Unfortunately, for many of us, unrelenting chronic stress is a sad fact of life. Surveys commissioned by the American Psychological Association have concluded that about 25 percent of us live with high levels of stress (that's an 8 on a 10-point scale) on a daily basis. Another 50 percent of us report having moderate levels of daily stress. It's no wonder—in 21st-century America, we're subject to a 24/7 news cycle that focuses on one horrific calamity after another. It's certainly easy to see how we all absorb way more than our share of worrisome messages.[1] And in these still-shaky economic times, many of us have burdensome worries about our job security and finances.

Stress Response 101

You're familiar with the fight-or-flight response. That's what nature gave our Paleo ancestors as a survival mechanism. It begins in the brain. When you confront danger (these days, the terrible driver instead of the saber-toothed tiger), your eyes and ears send the information to your brain's processing center, called the amygdala. When the amygdala registers danger, it shoots an SOS to the hypothalamus, your brain's central command. Its job is to send signals, via the autonomic nervous system, to trigger responses that help you deal with whatever crisis confronts you.

The command center also signals the adrenal glands to start pumping adrenaline throughout your system. This ramps up your heartbeat so that blood—and energy—can flow into your muscles, heart, and other vital organs. Up go your pulse and blood pressure. Your blood vessels widen or narrow, depending on your need (if you've been wounded, for example, your vessels would constrict to stem blood loss). Your breathing speeds up so your lungs and brain get more oxygen. Now, you're in a state of heightened alertness. You can hear and see more sharply, and you're better equipped to manage whatever challenge you're facing.

And, by the way, you're more or less unaware that this miracle of nature is occurring, because it happens nearly instantaneously. That's why you're able to swerve and slam on the brakes before you even perceive that car coming at you head-on.[2] This is some amazing system we're blessed with—miraculous, even. You can probably recall a time or two when your stress response actually saved your life or helped you avoid danger.

But when your miraculous stress response gets stuck in the "on" position and continually pumps adrenaline and other stress hormones throughout your body, that's when you run into trouble.

Sara's Stress Story

My coauthor, Sara Altshul, recently experienced what happens when stress spirals out of control, and she shared her story with me. Within months of each other, death claimed two beloved sisters-in-law. Then, budget cuts vaporized her husband's teaching position. A magazine job she loved came to an end, and a couple of other writing projects dried up.

Then, out of the blue, Sara's left knee started to hurt, but she ignored the pain—so much else was going on that needed her attention. Then she developed a nasty case of shingles. Now, in addition to her knee pain, she felt as if sharp, hot needles were tattooing her right flank.

Trust me, nothing good ever comes from ignoring your body when it's desperately trying to tell you something important. Pain is one way your body gets your attention.

Sara finally learned she had a torn meniscus (the cushion that surrounds the knee), complicated by a renegade bone shard. The answer was arthroscopic surgery to mend the meniscus and remove the fragment. She had the procedure, but a few days later, the pain was fiercer than ever. It was eye-popping pain. And guess what? She acquired *another* case of shingles, and this bout was even more painful than the first.

Her doctors were sympathetic and prescribed opioids to help her cope with the pain. What an imperfect solution that was! All she got was mushiness where her brain used to be. Her attention-getting sharp pains didn't disappear; they simply became dull, throbbing aches.

Finally, she'd had it. She asked me if there was anything she could do. I advised that she try water exercise and acupuncture. So Sara signed up for a 4-day-a-week aqua aerobics and aqua Zumba program at the Y. She also found a great acupuncturist and began weekly treatments. Additionally, I recommended that she take curcumin and fish oil supplements to deal with the inflammation. Happily, the pain started easing after just 2 weeks. I'm convinced the pool work and the acupuncture blunted her stress response, which, by the way, is proven to increase pain levels. The supplements eased the inflammation. What's more, those gentle water exercises were also great for strengthening her knee muscles, and acupuncture is proven to relieve pain (it has been extensively studied for knee pain relief). She stopped taking those narcotic pain pills.

Of course, Sara's stress didn't vaporize; but now that she didn't hurt so much, she could feel more hopeful about dealing with its causes.

Stress—It Does a Body Bad

Scientists have been scrutinizing the connections between stress and disease for at least 80 years. Back in 1936, Hans Selye, the pioneering stress researcher, defined stress as a "general adaptation syndrome" and believed that people experience physical reactions to various "noxious environmental agents." By the mid-1970s, the notion that stress could actually trigger chronic illness was gaining serious traction. That's when scientists began to identify the key stressors that they believed could heighten a person's susceptibility to disease. (Among them, two major stressors are clearly illustrated in Sara's story—bereavement and job loss.)[3]

Cut to the present. That stress plays a role in disease creation is pretty much common knowledge these days. But two recent studies shed light on two paths by which stress influences disease and health. And they are fascinating.

It turns out that there's a direct link between stress and inflammation, say researchers at Carnegie Mellon University (CMU) in Pittsburgh. In their 2012 study, they learned that when you're under chronic psychological stress, your body seems to lose its ability to control the inflammatory response. "Inflammation is partly regulated by the hormone cortisol," says Sheldon Cohen, PhD, the Robert E. Doherty Professor of Psychology at CMU's Dietrich College of Humanities and Social Sciences. Dr. Cohen goes on to explain that when you're under chronic stress, cortisol pumps out continually. Cells consistently subjected to this "cortisol waterfall" begin to lose their sensitivity to the hormone.

Among the cells that become insensitive to cortisol are the immune cells, which are supposed to keep disease-causing elements away. Since insensitive immune cells are ineffective immune cells, that's how runaway inflammation can promote the development and progression of many diseases.[4]

Dr. Cohen, by the way, is no stranger to studying the effects of stress on the human body. Back in 1991, in his landmark *New England Journal of Medicine* study, he gave 394 healthy adults questionnaires to measure their stress levels.[5] His team then administered nose drops to them that contained various common cold viruses. He quarantined them all for 5 days and monitored them for signs of infection. The participants developed colds at rates that matched their stress levels. Nearly half of the most stressed-out people developed colds, while only 27 percent of people experiencing less stress got sick.

Over the years, studies have shown that chronic psychological stress actually alters DNA, which could explain why stress makes some people more susceptible to chronic disease. But in a 2012 study, researchers discovered that even *fleeting* stress (as you might experience during a job interview, for example) could change DNA in a way that might promote chronic disease. "Epigenetic changes may well be an important link between stress and chronic diseases," says lead author Gunther Meinlschmidt, professor and head of the research department of psychobiology, psychosomatics, and psychotherapy at the LWL University Hospital of Rurh University in Bochum, Germany. He and his team of European researchers noted that complex epigenetic stress patterns would be the target of future study.[6]

Tapping into Antistress Strategies

Dealing with the two kinds of stress we encounter—chronic and acute—means you need to set aside time to practice the techniques proven to keep stress at bay. Just as you're weaving a new way of eating into your life and learning how to become more active, you also need to make conscious stress relief part of your daily plan. In this chapter, I'll outline some of the most scientifically tested and trusted stress-busting methods available. When you add these to your No More Pills eating and activity programs, you'll be doing all you can to help keep chronic diseases—and pills—out of your life.

Tap Your Way to Stress Relief

When it comes to dealing with acute stress, one therapy I recommend time and time again is called the *emotional freedom technique* (EFT). It's a deceptively simple, scientifically studied self-healing tool that takes minutes to learn and can often provide quick and lasting relief for both acute and chronic stress.

EFT evolved from a practice called *thought field therapy,* which was developed in the early 1980s by a clinical psychologist named Roger Callahan.

Thought field therapy was simplified a decade later by Dr. Callahan's student Gary Craig, a Stanford graduate engineer.[7] In EFT, you tap with fingertip pressure on a set pattern of acupressure points. As you tap, you murmur a phrase—an intention—that focuses you and helps you counter your current stress in a positive way. Though it sounds fairly incredible, this exercise lowers your body's stress response and even makes changes in old neurologic patterns, notably in severe post-traumatic stress disorder (PTSD).[8] There are now many good studies, including a number of studies done with veterans suffering from PTSD, documenting the effectiveness of EFT.

According to Mark Hyman, MD, who recently opened the Center for Functional Medicine at the Cleveland Clinic, EFT's "tapping interrupts the body's stress response quickly and effectively." In his foreword to *The Tapping Solution*, a book by renowned EFT expert Nick Ortner, Dr. Hyman writes that tapping is a "fast-acting, noninvasive way to proactively manage the stress that so often leaves our bodies vulnerable to disease."[9]

Doing the EFT Tapping

Follow these simple steps, and pretty soon, the EFT exercise will become second nature to you. You'll be able to perform it anytime you need to ease your response to a stressful situation.

1. **Put your worry into words.** First, choose the one issue that's most troubling for you. It could be a stressful deadline, a money worry, a persistent ache or pain, or a work problem. Turn it into a short phrase, such as "My knee is killing me" or "I'm so upset about the mistake I made at work." The point is to describe exactly what's bothering you. As one of my EFT mentors, Alina Frank, says, "Make it specific."

2. **Rate how troubled you are.** On a scale of 0 to 10, rank the level of anxiety this concern causes you. Be aware of that level as you move through the exercise. This is called "SUDS" level (subjective units of distress).

3. **Craft a phrase.** In EFT language, this is called a set-up statement. Here's a basic one from Ortner in *The Tapping Solution*. "Even

Don's Story

I've used EFT successfully to help many people overcome stress-linked problems, but one patient I learned about in my EFT studies is particularly unforgettable. This story comes from EFT coach Ingrid Dinter.

Don* is a 61-year-old Vietnam War veteran who has Parkinson's disease. He worked with therapist Dinter for a total of 6 EFT session hours. Since returning from Vietnam, Don hadn't experienced a single night of uninterrupted sleep. He never slept more than a couple of hours at a stretch, and never more than 4 to 5 hours a night. Even worse, horrific nightmares woke him at least twice a night.

His first session took only 20 minutes; it was all Don could handle that day. Before starting with EFT, he told Dinter his thoughts were like bumper cars, bouncing all over, but the tapping helped him relax and release the tension in his mind. It also stopped the Parkinson's tremors and shaking. The therapist helped him tap on finding peace with the war and peace with Vietnam. After this brief first session, his sleep greatly improved: He now slept 6 to 7 hours, woke up twice briefly, and felt rested instead of fatigued.

In each of the subsequent sessions, Dinter worked through several traumatic war-related memories with Don. She released his sadness and guilt using the gentle EFT techniques and tapped on deserving forgiveness.

By the end of his therapy, Don was going to bed between 9:45 and 10:15, was sleeping 7 to 8 hours, and had no more nightmares. Reviewing his progress, Don said, "I still think about Vietnam, but it doesn't seem to bother me." He continues to tap on his Parkinson's symptoms to keep the shaking under control. His wife has noticed that he seems happier and relaxed, Dinter reported. He feels comfortable socializing now and is a true believer in EFT.[10]

*Name changed

though I'm anxious and fearful about how much <u>my knee hurts</u>, I deeply and completely accept myself." (You fill in the underlined part with your particular concern.)[11]

4. **Assess your SUDS level** with a specific number, even if it's just a guesstimate.

5. **Start tapping.** Now you can actually begin tapping. To start, say your set-up statement out loud three times. As you do this, take two fingers and tap on the "karate chop" point of your other hand. This is where the top crease in your palm ends, right below your pinkie.

6. **Tapping the reminder statement.** After repeating the setup statement three times, you are ready to go on to the reminder statement. As an example, a reminder statement would be: "The anxiety and fear about the pain in my knee . . . " Start tapping at the crown of your head, and tap several times at each of these points. You can tap with just one hand on one side or use both hands. Here are the points:

- Crown of the head
- Inner edge of eyebrow
- Outer side of the eye
- Middle of the space below the nose and above the upper lip
- Middle of the chin below the lower lip
- Just below the "knobs" of the collarbone
- Just below the armpit

After you have tapped through all the points, stop, take a deep breath, and reassess your SUDS level. Repeat the process until you have reached a level of 2, 1, or 0. If you have trouble or your stress increases, consider getting some help. Many certified EFT practitioners do Skype and phone sessions, or you could visit one in person.

These instructions are a very brief outline of the EFT process. For more information, download the free EFT mini-manual from eftuniverse.com, and try a few coaching sessions with a certified EFT practitioner.

Refocusing Emotion to Blunt Stress

A while back, I learned about a wonderful system called HeartMath, whose mission is to help people reduce stress and increase their emotional balance. The rationale behind the program's techniques is that you can "learn how to neutralize and counter the effects of stress by actively adding a positive feeling such as appreciation, care, and compassion to the process," say the HeartMath experts. They believe that you can experience positive emotions by generating feelings of appreciation, care, or compassion—and that doing so can help you manage your stress.

In particular, I use and recommend one of their techniques, called Freeze-Frame, developed by one of HeartMath's founders, Rollin McCraty, PhD, a psychologist and renowned stress expert. Dr. McCraty and his team have helped corporate CEOs, medical professionals, athletes, performers, and even police and the military reduce their stress levels via HeartMath programs.

There are five steps to Freeze-Frame.

1. **Recognize** . . . that you're feeling stress and take a time-out so you can put your feelings and thoughts on hold.

2. **Shift** . . . your focus to the area of your heart. Now breathe in as if your breath is flowing in through the center of your chest and out through your stomach area. Practice breathing this way to ease into the technique. Breathe in for 4 to 5 seconds and then breathe out for 4 to 5 seconds. Breathe quietly and naturally. Continue this rhythmic breathing as you do the rest of the steps.

3. **Activate** . . . a positive feeling. This can be a genuine feeling of appreciation or caring for someone, some place (your favorite beach or hiking trail, for example), or something wonderful in your life. It's important to actually feel the feeling this thought engenders.

4. **Ask** . . . yourself what would be a better way to handle this situation or what action would reduce your stress. Try to select a less stressful perspective, even if you can't feel it yet.

5. **Notice** . . . any change in the way you think and feel about the situation. Try to remember any new thoughts and feelings for as long as you can.[12]

For more information, visit heartmath.com.

Guided Imagery

Guided imagery is an excellent way to relax and reduce stress. It uses words and music to bring positive images into your mind.

I can't say enough about the effectiveness and wonderful calming qualities of guided imagery and its leading practitioner and advocate, Belleruth Naparstek. Thanks mainly to her smiling, dedicated energy, guided imagery is now one of the best-studied mind-body methods we have. Naparstek's guided imagery CDs and MP3 downloads have helped countless people with surgery and surgical recovery, anxiety, sleep problems, trauma, fertility, weight loss, and many other issues. In guided imagery, you only need to find a quiet place (not behind the wheel, please) and listen to the program. Visit her Web site for research and stress relief programs at healthjourneys.com.

How Compassion Calms You Down

In a similar vein to the HeartMath approach is the much more ancient technique called self-compassion. Its kindred concept is practicing compassion for everyone—including compassion toward people who actively get your goat or actually do you wrong, deliberately or not. Although compassion has its roots in Buddhist tradition, its practice is absolutely nondenominational; I view it as mindfulness. I've found one particular practice, called *metta bhavana,* to be especially helpful for relieving stressful feelings, especially after a long day of caring for patients. You might also find it really helpful after a full day of office meetings, for example.

Proving the point that compassion can lead to calmer feelings, a 2014 study published in *Health Psychology* investigated the health benefits of self-compassion. The study looked at 3,252 records that linked compassion with a set of health-promoting behaviors. The researchers concluded that self-compassion could actually help promote healthy behaviors.[13]

So what does this mean for you? We asked one of the study's authors, Jameson K. Hirsch, PhD, associate professor in East Tennessee State University's department of psychology, to explain. First of all, he says, being mindful is key to reaping the health benefits of compassion. "Understanding that others are in similar or even worse situations than you are, and then being mindful of your pain, discomfort, stress, or fears, rather than ignoring them or worrying about them, is an important outcome of practicing mindfulness," he adds.

In his studies, Dr. Hirsch and his team learned that self-compassion was linked to healthy behaviors, such as exercising and eating right, and they also learned that the more people practiced self-compassion, the more they also practiced these beneficial behaviors. What's more, the researchers learned that self-compassion improves your mood—and the better your mood, the more likely you'll be "kind" to yourself by exercising more or eating healthier foods, says Dr. Hirsch. "It may also be the case that self-compassion allows you to effectively cope with the setbacks that often accompany working toward your health goals, so that if you mess up on your diet or miss a workout, it will be easier for you to get back on track," says Dr. Hirsch. That's because practicing self-compassion means you're not so hard on yourself, so it's easier to forgive yourself when you slip and to get back to your program the next day.

So back to *metta bhavana*. The word *metta* means nonromantic love, which translates to friendliness or kindness. That's why the Buddhists refer to it as loving-kindness. You feel loving-kindness in your heart, says the Buddhist tradition. The word *bhavana* refers to the practice part of this exercise: It means cultivation. I learned to practice *metta bhavana* in six stages.

Here's how to get started. The entire exercise should take you about 5 minutes.

1. **Focus on you.** Start by becoming aware of yourself, and focus on feelings of peace, calm, and tranquility.

2. **Feel confidence and love.** Let yourself feel strength and confidence, and then develop that into a feeling of love within your heart. You can use an image, like golden light flooding your body, or a phrase such as "May I be well and happy," which you can repeat to yourself. These are ways of stimulating the feeling of *metta* for yourself.

3. **Think of a good friend.** Bring this person to mind as vividly as you can and think of her good qualities. Feel your connection with your friend and your liking for her, and encourage these to grow by repeating "May she be well; may she be happy" quietly to yourself.

4. **Think of someone neutral.** This may be someone you do not know well but see around. Reflect on his humanity and include him in your feelings of *metta*. Now return to yourself and repeat "May I be well and happy."

5. **Think of someone you actually dislike.** Here's the challenging part: Don't get caught up in your feelings of hatred; instead, think of this positively and send your *metta* to him, as well.

6. **Finally, think of all four people together.** Think of yourself, your friend, your neutral person, and your enemy. Then extend your feelings further, to everyone around you—to everyone in your neighborhood, in your town, in your country, and so on throughout the world. Have a sense of waves of loving-kindness spreading out from you.

Now, don't you feel calmer and more relaxed? Of course you do.[14]

Breathing Stress Away

Rhythmic breathing, or "breath work," is a stress-relieving practice used in many complementary healing practices, including traditional Chinese medicine and Ayurveda, the traditional medicine of India. According to Andrew Weil, MD, the father of integrative medicine, "Practicing regular, mindful breathing can be calming and energizing, and can even help with stress-related health problems ranging from panic attacks to digestive disorders." Among the stress-relieving breathing techniques Dr. Weil recommends frequently is one called the 4-7-8 Breathing Exercise (also called the Relaxing Breath).

You can practice this exercise anywhere, and it takes just a few minutes to learn. Commit it to memory and you'll have a tool to calm you down even in the heat of the most stressful times.

You can do 4-7-8 in any position, but while you're learning, Dr. Weil recommends that you sit down, keeping your back nice and straight. Place the tip of your tongue against the ridge of tissue behind your upper front teeth, and keep it there throughout the exercise. You will exhale through your mouth around your tongue. If it's easier for you, purse your lips slightly.

1. Exhale completely through your mouth, making a whooshing sound.

2. Close your mouth and inhale quietly through your nose to a mental count of four.

3. Hold your breath while silently counting to seven.

4. Exhale completely through your mouth, making a whooshing sound, to a silent count of eight.

5. This is one breath. Now, inhale again and repeat the cycle three more times for a total of four breaths.[15]

Achieving the Relaxation Response

One of the longest-studied approaches to managing stress is something called the relaxation response. Herbert Benson, MD, associate professor of medicine at Harvard Medical School and cofounder, along with Joan Borysenko, PhD, of the Mind/Body Medical Institute in Chestnut Hill, Massachusetts, coined this term in the early 1970s. He essentially observed people who did breath meditation and studied the physiology of their responses. Dr. Benson has dedicated his career to teaching and researching how the relaxation response counters the harmful effects of stress.

The relaxation response is what happens to your body when you meditate or employ other stress-relieving techniques. As Dr. Benson learned through his many studies, when you meditate or engage in other mind-body relaxation practices, your body produces physical changes. You consume less oxygen, and your breathing slows. Chemical stress markers in your blood decrease. Your blood pressure goes down, and you begin to feel more peaceful and contented. Couldn't you use a little more peace and contentment in your life?[16]

In his landmark book, *The Relaxation Response,* Dr. Benson outlined the steps for triggering a physical state of calm that counters stress. He shares it on his Web site at relaxationresponse.org. It is basically a combination of progressive relaxation techniques commonly used in hypnosis—tensing, then relaxing the muscles—plus simple breath meditation. Here's how to practice this meditative technique.

1. Sit quietly in a comfortable position.

2. Close your eyes.

3. Deeply relax all your muscles, slowly, beginning at your feet and progressing up to your face. Keep your muscles relaxed throughout the exercise.

4. Breathe through your nose. Become aware of your breathing. As you breathe out, say the word "one" (or any soothing, mellifluous sound, preferably one with no meaning—you don't want to stimulate unnecessary thoughts) silently to yourself. Breathe easily and naturally.

5. Continue for 10 to 20 minutes. You may open your eyes to check the time, but don't use an alarm. When you're finished, sit quietly for several minutes, first with your eyes closed, then with your eyes open.

6. Don't worry about whether you're "successful" in achieving a deep state of relaxation. Maintain a passive attitude and permit relaxation to occur at its own pace. When distracting thoughts flutter into your mind, don't dwell on them; return to repeating your word.

According to Dr. Benson, you should be able to achieve the relaxation response easily. Practice the exercise once or twice a day—but not within 2 hours after eating, since the digestive process seems to interfere with bringing on the response.[17]

Find What Works for You

Some of these strategies are likely to resonate better with you than others, so pick the ones that feel most natural. Set aside some time each day to practice—10 to 20 minutes once or twice a day is ideal. Put your stress relief time in your calendar, and don't let anything get in the way of your practice. In just a few weeks, if not sooner, you'll notice that you feel calmer and more centered and that the little things that once made you tense aren't quite so alarming anymore. That's the whole point! Just remember that some people might have difficulty with some—even all—of these methods. Sometimes, if you have unresolved trauma, or are just a very high-energy person, sitting and trying to relax may end up being too much "trying" and not relaxing at all. In fact, if you're this kind of person, sitting quietly may even make you feel more anxious. If that's true for you, pick some other activity that feels relaxing. For you, it may be running, yoga, listening to music, or even reading a book. If you feel even more tense when you're trying to relax or you have unresolved trauma, consider working with a certified EFT practitioner with trauma expertise.

Of course, you don't need to practice each of these antistress techniques every day, but I would like to see you take 10 to 20 minutes daily to practice some form of calming activity. The more stress you have in your life, the longer you should focus on activities that will mitigate its effects on your body.

Part II

Your Condition-Specific Protocol

Allergies

Allergies come in many varieties, and though the causes and symptoms may differ, one thing is certain—allergies are on the rise, and their symptoms can make you miserable. Something like 50 million Americans report having an allergy of one kind or another, and even the country's leading medical group for allergy specialists admits that we don't fully understand why some people have allergies or why some substances commonly trigger uncomfortable symptoms.[1]

In Chapter 2, I talked about the fact that our increasingly toxic environment assaults our immune systems with substances they were never designed to process, including food additives; genetically modified foods; pesticides; chemicals from cleaning solutions, cosmetics, and many other products; and pharmaceuticals, traces of which are now widely found in our water systems. In my opinion, and in the opinion of many integrative physicians like me, these and other environmental insults have put our immune systems on high alert so that they are more reactive here in the 21st century than ever before. This, I believe, explains why statistics show that allergies are on the rise.

In Chapter 2, I discussed the kinds of problems that food allergies can cause. In this section, I'm going to discuss allergy symptoms caused by airborne particles (I'll collectively call them allergens) such as pollen, dust mites, and mold spores—and how to ease those symptoms with the No More Pills Plan.

Why Am I Sneezing?

Blame it on your immune system. When you're allergic to something, such as pollen, your immune system goes on high alert and produces antibodies called immunoglobulin E (IgE). Different types of IgE activate for different allergens. That's why some people might be allergic only to pollen from certain trees, while others react to ragweed or grass pollens, and still other people react only to cat dander or mold spores, for example. A number of extremely sensitive people may react to several different allergens.

What's My Problem?

Since the symptoms of allergies, colds, and sinusitis can be similar, you may not know which problem you have or how best to treat yourself. Here's how to spot the differences among these common problems.

Probably an allergy if . . .

You have a runny or stuffy nose, sneezing, wheezing, and watery or itchy eyes.

Symptoms begin shortly after exposure to an allergen.

Symptoms abate once you're away from the allergen.

Probably a cold or flu if . . .

In addition to allergy symptoms, you also have a sore throat, body aches, and fever.

Symptoms develop over a few days.

Symptoms clear up in less than a week. Flu recovery might take a little longer.

Probably sinusitis if . . .

You have a headache or swollen feeling around your forehead, eyes, and cheeks; a stuffy nose with thick, colored mucus; bad-tasting postnasal drip; bad breath; sore throat; and cough, fatigue, and low fever.

Symptoms linger. Acute sinusitis symptoms could last for a month. Chronic sinusitis lasts 3 months or longer.[2]

When triggered, the IgE antibodies shoot to cells that release chemicals called histamines. These are what cause the respiratory symptoms. Some people also experience eye sensitivity called allergic conjunctivitis, when eyes react by swelling, reddening, and watering when a sensitive person comes in contact with an allergen. Still other people may experience hives, itching, or other skin reactions to allergens.[3, 4]

Hay fever is the common term for seasonal allergies caused when trees, weeds, and grasses release tiny pollen grains into the air—no matter what the actual season. If you're allergic to the pollens you inhale, you'll react with a runny or clogged nose; coughing and postnasal drip; itchy eyes, nose, and throat; and even dark circles under your eyes.

Some physicians diagnose hay fever after giving you a physical and hearing about your symptoms. Sometimes, a physician will recommend skin or blood tests to determine what's causing your symptoms.

And of course, many, if not most, doctors will prescribe pills—an antihistamine of some sort or one of the steroid-based nasal sprays, or both.

Side Effects of Allergy Meds

Let's take pseudoephedrine (Sudafed), the popular decongestant, for starters. Though you can buy it over the counter in any drugstore, it's actually a stimulant that can raise your blood pressure and cause a variety of cardiac side effects. And if you're a *Breaking Bad* fan, you'll remember that pseudoephedrine is one of the ingredients druggies use to concoct homemade methamphetamine—that's why most drugstores have it under lock and key these days. Interestingly, when herbal supplements (often, a weight loss product) make headlines for causing fatal or serious side effects, it turns out that most of those supplements contain the herb ephedra or the ephedra compound ephedrine. This compound is nearly identical to pseudoephedrine (the word actually means "fake ephedrine," for heaven's sake) in Sudafed. Which, as I already mentioned, is sold over the counter, though you're limited as to how much you can purchase at a time.

In addition, those corticosteroid inhalers that doctors so often prescribe for allergies have been linked to causing osteoporosis. I also believe they can lower your immunity and increase the risk of nasal and sinus infections.[5]

Older antihistamines, such as diphenhydramine (Benadryl), for example, can make you drowsy—so drowsy that driving or doing anything else that requires your complete attention may be impaired. Newer drugs, such as fexofenadine (Allegra), may cause side effects that include cough or stomach upset.[6]

You Don't Have to Move

At one time, physicians treating people with severe allergies or asthma might have given their patients the conventional wisdom of the day, which was to suggest they move to a dry, desert-type environment like Arizona, where they'd supposedly be less likely to encounter pollen and other allergens. But now we know that moving might not be so helpful after all. The largest, most comprehensive study ever conducted on the prevalence of allergies from early childhood to old age was published in 2014 in the *Journal of Clinical Immunology*. It analyzed data compiled from blood tests of some 10,000 Americans who were part of the National Health and Nutrition Examination Study (NHANES) in 2005 to 2006. The research showed that people who are prone to developing allergies are likely to develop an allergy to whatever is in their environment, no matter where they live, says Darryl Zeldin, MD, scientific director of the National Institute of Environmental Health Sciences.[7, 8] So, allergy sufferers, you can rest easy and stay put, unless, of course, you live close to a coal-fired power plant, for example, or some other obvious source of pollution.

The No More Pills Antiallergy Rx

Before you go the prescription or over-the-counter pill route to seek an allergy remedy, I have a number of suggestions that can make managing your symptoms much easier—and they won't require you to live in a plastic bubble during allergy season!

Tweak Your No More Pills Plan
During Allergy Season

The good news is that the No More Pills Plan will benefit people with allergies because it features foods that help reduce inflammation in our bodies. Why is this so important?

Here's your answer: When people who are allergic to pollens or other allergens come in contact with them, it sets off an internal cascade of inflammatory reactions, which in turn create troublesome symptoms. So what you really don't want to do, in essence, is add fuel to the fire by eating foods that also create internal inflammation. Inflammatory foods can worsen pollen and other airborne allergies for some people and include dairy, wheat, processed foods, food additives and colorings, nonorganic and non-grass-fed red meats, trans fats, and sugary foods, for example.

On the other hand, eating foods rich in anti-inflammatory compounds will, especially over time, support your body in ways that can help lower your allergic reactions. Interestingly, researchers actually proved this theory back in a 2007 study conducted with 690 children, 7 to 18 years of age, on the Mediterranean island of Crete.

The research team discovered that 80 percent of the kids they surveyed (via their parents) ate fresh fruit and 68 percent ate vegetables at least twice a day. Primarily, those fruits and veggies were Crete's local produce—grapes, oranges, apples, and fresh tomatoes. Turns out, eating those foods seemed to help protect the kids against wheezing and pollen-type allergy symptoms—sneezing, runny nose, and the like. What's more, eating nuts was also linked to less wheezing, and for what it's worth, eating margarine (which you certainly won't be eating on the No More Pills Plan) actually *increased* the children's allergy symptoms.[9]

Eat these foods more often:

- Dark green, leafy veggies
- Deep yellow and orange veggies
- Onions, garlic, ginger, cayenne, horseradish
- Wild and organic fish, which contain plenty of anti-inflammatory omega-3 fatty acids
- Plenty of pure water—drink half your body weight in ounces every day (for a 150-pound person, that's 75 ounces of water)[10, 11]

Avoid these totally:

- Dairy
- Wheat
- Corn
- Processed foods
- Food additives and dyes

Allergy-Proof Your Home

Your home should be a safe sanctuary—not a place that makes your allergies even worse than they already are. So removing allergens from your indoor atmosphere is essential. I recommend installing air filters, either free-standing ones or filters that are installed in your home's heating and cooling system. I prefer HEPA filters that use charcoal/zeolite to remove airborne chemicals, and I particularly like filters that use UV light. A good (though somewhat pricey) brand is AllerAir. These are made of metal, rather than plastic, which can emit unhealthy gases; they can cost up to $1,000. A cheaper but very effective filter is the Surround Air filter. It uses UV light and has a HEPA-charcoal filter that needs to be replaced every 3 to 4 months.

I have AllerAir *and* Surround Air filters in both my home and office, and these have greatly improved my air quality.

If you're allergic to dust mites or mold spores, you want to make sure your indoor atmosphere is as clear of these irritants as possible. Here's how.

- Frequently vacuum (with a HEPA-filter machine) and shampoo carpets.

- Remove your shoes at the door and slip into house slippers once you're inside.

- Clean your home furnace vents regularly and use a high-quality furnace filter.

- Use blinds instead of curtains at your windows and clean them regularly.

- Cover your pillows and mattress with dust mite covers.[12]

Another trick to keeping your immune system from overreacting to allergens is to rinse them away as soon as you can. So take a shower and shampoo your hair as soon as you can after you've been out and about during allergy season.

Also, don't pollute your indoor environment by using plug-in or spray air fresheners, or scented candles. And avoid using toxic cleaning products. I've seen so many allergies and illnesses caused by household chemicals that we could devote an entire book to this subject.

Reach for This Herb

Butterbur (*Petasites vulgaris*) is a large-leafed European herb that was nicknamed "plague flower" because it was once a remedy for bubonic plague. Its tradition as a healing herb stretches back to the 17th century as a remedy for respiratory problems. Modern science confirms what early herbalists knew: Butterbur can alleviate allergies. In a 2002 *British Medical Journal* study, conducted in four Swiss and German clinics, 125 hay fever sufferers were split into two groups. One received butterbur extract; the other took the prescription antihistamine cetirizine (Zyrtec). After 2 weeks, both treatments were equally effective at relieving symptoms.[13] A few years later, in 2005, the same research team compared butterbur extract to the prescription antihistamine fexofenadine (Allegra). They assigned 330 people to one of three groups: One group took butterbur extract, another group took fexofenadine, and the third group was given a placebo. The butterbur and the antihistamine relieved allergy symptoms equally effectively, and both treatments beat the placebo.[14]

Butterbur contains compounds called petasines, which hinder the activity of compounds called leukotrienes, part of the body's immune system response that triggers allergy symptoms. The extract used in the studies is Petadolex. Take one capsule three times a day.[15]

Vitamins and Other Supplements

I rely on four key supplements to ease nasty allergy symptoms. These all play a role in helping your body lessen its reaction to allergens.

Vitamin C is considered a natural antihistamine. Though the research is mixed, some studies have shown that taking 2,000 milligrams of vitamin C a day can ease allergy symptoms.[16]

Bioflavonoids (including quercetin, catechin, and hesperidin) are antioxidants that are also natural antihistamines and strongly antiallergenic. Quercetin comes from apples, onions, and tea (among other foods). Catechins are found in green tea, and hesperidin is found in citrus fruit.

You can find combination bioflavonoid supplements; take 2 to 3 grams a day.[17, 18]

Probiotics also lower allergic reactivity by balancing the gut ecosystem and helping to lower inflammation. My favorite is Renew Life Ultimate Flora, which comes in several strengths and is widely available. I take a 50-billion capsule every day, and I've been using it with hundreds of patients over several years now with great results. It has a good combination of beneficial bacteria, and it's convenient to travel with because it doesn't need to be refrigerated. (Of course, you don't want to keep it in your hot car, but room temperature is fine.)

Vitamin E might calm your immune system's reaction to allergens and lessen your symptoms, though the evidence isn't overwhelming. In one 2004 study, 112 people with hay fever were given either 800 IU of vitamin E or a placebo for 10 weeks. They also continued to take their antiallergy medications during the study, and researchers recorded the amounts of pills they took. Those in the vitamin E group reported having significantly fewer nasal symptoms—particularly stuffiness—than people in the control group.[19]

Worth a Try: Homeopathy

Homeopathy is a more than 200-year-old practice that admittedly is tricky to explain to anyone who is rooted in conventional Western medicine.

The principle behind this "less is more" modality is that practitioners use substances that might cause symptoms in a healthy person to cure those symptoms in a sick person. But these remedies are extremely diluted— in fact, they might not contain a single molecule of the original medicine. Using these dilute remedies, say homeopathic physicians, somehow stimulates the body's self-healing mechanisms. One parallel that conventional medicine shares with homeopathy: If you take allergy desensitization shots, you're getting inoculated with a tiny amount of the allergen that provokes your symptoms.[20]

When you are considering homeopathy, it's important to remember its history. Homeopathy earned its stripes in Europe by being effective against epidemics of typhus and cholera. According to medical records of doctors at that time, during several cholera epidemics, the mortality rate of patients who were given homeopathic remedies was only 9 percent, slightly less than

1 in 10. The mortality rate of people given conventional allopathic treatment was 40 to 80 percent.

Another observation about homeopathy is this: There is a homeopathic pharmacy on "every other block" in France and Germany. These are some of the most scientific and medically sophisticated countries in the world. I absolutely have no idea why they would maintain a whole medical system if it didn't work. The reason why we do not have homeopathy here in the United States is that it was deliberately drummed out of town by the competing allopathic system.

No gold standard–type, randomized, controlled clinical trials exist to prove exactly how effective homeopathic allergy treatment might be. Part of the reason for that is that in classical homeopathy, treatment is individualized to the patient, so comparisons in a medical study are difficult to make. However, a couple of studies do point to homeopathy's potential benefit for people with allergies.

In a 2013 study published in the journal *Homeopathy*, researchers recruited 30 people with known allergies to cats. They assigned 15 people for treatments with two homeopathic medications: Cat saliva 9cH and Histaminum 9cH; the other 15 people got a placebo. After 4 weeks, the homeopathic remedy reduced allergic reactions significantly; people in the placebo group were unaffected.[21]

In a 2012 Austrian study, when 40 people with allergies were treated with classical homeopathy along with their allergy medications, 62 percent were able to discontinue at least one of their allergy drugs, and 38 percent were able to reduce the dosage of at least one of their medications.[22]

I recommend common homeopathic remedies for allergies, such as the Boiron Optique 1 allergy eye drops. I practically cured my inhalant allergies just by using them two to four times a day during allergy season, and I have had very good results with many patients as well. They are very safe to use and to carry around. They come in sealed sterile plastic dropper vials. You just twist off the top and squeeze half the sterile liquid into each eye, drop by drop.

Sometimes I will refer people to a good homeopath for complicated allergy problems, especially if they're committed to having homeopathy be their major treatment over quite a period of time. You can find a registered homeopath at homeopathy.org.

● ●

DR. HOWARD'S Q&A

Q. I've tested positive to certain trees that spew pollen in the spring. I love to be outdoors, but this ruins it for me. What can I do?

A. First of all, make sure your indoor space is pollen-free by running the air conditioner and keeping windows closed. This may sound tough to do, but if you aren't also being exposed to pollens circulating inside your house, you'll have less trouble when you are outside. Also, consider seeing a good allergist for desensitization drops or shots.

Arthritis

The experts at the Arthritis Foundation list 21 different diseases on the foundation's Arthritis A–Z Web page.[1] But by far the most common form of this wear-and-tear disease is osteoarthritis (OA), which affects some 27 million Americans. That's because this painful condition occurs when the cartilage that cushions your joints begins to wear out and tear down, and as a result, your bones start rubbing against each other. Just thinking about that scenario is enough to make your joints ache.[2]

The sad truth is, there's no cure for OA. Its symptoms develop slowly, over time. In the beginning, you'll probably think of your newly discovered aches and pains as something that's not such a big deal—until a few years or more later, when they really start getting your attention. The all-too-familiar symptoms can include:

- Sore, stiff joints, especially after inactivity

- Stiffness after resting that disappears with movement

- Pain that worsens after activity or at day's end

You can experience arthritis pain in any joint, but arthritis most commonly targets the hips, knees, and neck. You can also experience arthritis pain in your hands. X-ray evidence shows that the finger joints (the distal and proximal interphalangeal joints of the hand) are most often affected by osteoarthritis, but they don't generally cause a lot of pain.

As the months and years pass, especially under certain circumstances, those minor aches and pains can become activity-limiting pain. That's when you start thinking twice about engaging in treasured activities, such as playing tennis or hiking.

Fortunately, you've come to the right place to learn ways to lessen your arthritis pain. The key is to start now because following the No More Pills Plan at the earliest twinges of arthritis, or even before that, gives you your best shot at slowing the disease's progression and keeping your joints as pain-free as possible.[3]

Age Is Just One OA Factor

We used to think of osteoarthritis (derived from two Greek words meaning "bone" and "joint") as a condition that naturally comes with the territory of aging, one that few people are lucky enough to sidestep as they get older. But now we know better. Osteoarthritis is actually an umbrella term for several different subtypes of the disease based on different causes, agreed participants at a major Arthritis Foundation workshop held in Chicago in 2012.[4] Let's take a look at the triggers they've identified so far.

Genes. Researchers are particularly keen on unraveling the connection between genes and OA. Their work has led so far to the discovery of three genes linked to a higher predisposition for acquiring the disease; they continue to seek others. But, caution the experts, we're far from being able to say that certain OA genes lead *directly* to the disease—and even further away from being able to offer treatments. "The hope is, as we identify more OA susceptibility genes, we'll be able to offer new treatments," says John Loughlin, PhD, professor of musculoskeletal research at Newcastle University Musculoskeletal Group in England. In an interview with *Arthritis Today,* Dr. Loughlin, who is also secretary of the Osteoarthritis Research Society International, additionally noted that one day we might be able to help people predict their OA risk based on their genetic profile.[5]

Injury. One arthritis subtype, called post-traumatic OA, is caused by traumatic injuries to the hip, knee, or ankle. In fact, some 12 percent of the worst arthritis cases are triggered by an injury. Research now shows that 10 to 20 years after a traumatic knee injury, such as an ACL or meniscus tear, 50 percent of the injured people will develop OA.

Obesity. Being overweight can also lead to OA, and you don't need to be a physiology expert to understand why. When you put more pressure on joints than they're designed to handle, it stresses and compacts the cartilage cushion, causing it to degrade. But wait, there's more. Researchers now understand that fat tissue releases chemicals that increase inflammation, and that can wreak havoc on cartilage. Researchers have put one such chemical, the hormone leptin, under study. They've learned that higher leptin levels in fat tissue are directly related to the narrowing of joint space in the hip (an arthritis sign). In other studies, high blood levels of leptin paralleled high pain scores in people with OA.

Aging. Though it's clear that aging isn't the only factor that causes OA, it's still a significant one. Of course, if aging was OA's solo cause, then all senior-aged folks would develop it. And that's simply not the case at all.

Obesity, genetics, and injury all play a role in causing the disease, says Richard Loeser Jr., MD, distinguished professor of medicine in the division of rheumatology, allergy, and immunology and director of basic and translational research at the Thurston Arthritis Research Center at the University of North Carolina at Chapel Hill. "The age-related changes in the joint contribute to its development," he says. Which begs the question, so why don't we all have OA after a certain age? In a Dutch study of more than 80 people ages 89 to 91, 63 percent had arthritis-free hips, 51 percent didn't have arthritis in their knees, and 29 percent didn't have arthritis in their hands. So who made it to their golden years free of arthritis? People who tend to escape OA's clutches even into their eighties or nineties share these factors:

- They've maintained a normal weight.
- There's no family history of nodal arthritis of the hands (a type that tends to run in families).[6]
- They produce low levels of inflammatory compounds called interleukin proteins.
- They've performed heavy physical labor throughout much of their lives.

As Dr. Loeser explained to *Arthritis Today*, "The message we're trying to get out is that OA is not simply a degenerative disease of aging. It's an active, inflammatory disease. Your joints aren't like automobiles that wear out over time."[7]

The No More Pills Arthritis-Easing Rx

The sad truth is that conventional medicine has very little to offer people with OA except pills (nonsteroidal anti-inflammatory drugs, known as NSAIDs) with their worrisome side effects and surgery with limited effectiveness.[8, 9]

That's why the No More Pills Plan is such great news for you. It fuses diet, strategic supplement use, stress-relief techniques, and gentle movement to help you ease pain and loosen joints. Unlike taking NSAIDs that can seriously up your risk for heart attacks, strokes, and ulcers and bleeding in the stomach or intestines, or having surgery that might not relieve pain (and could cause its own unintended and negative consequences), the No More Pills Plan for OA means you'll learn how to maximize your body's ability to continue building cartilage—or at least not lose it as quickly. You'll also learn about acupuncture and how certain mind/body practices can help you relieve your pain. Let's start with diet.

The No More Pills Plan: Perfect for OA Pain

As much as I'd like to refrain from repeating certain truths time and time again in this book, I just can't help myself. Especially when it comes to the benefits of the No More Pills Plan for so many of the conditions we'll cover. Why is this? Because so much disease has underlying inflammation, and so much of that inflammation, in my opinion, is caused by inflammatory reactions to common foods. I created the No More Pills Plan specifically to be as anti-inflammatory as possible.

That said, some foods on the plan are extra helpful when it comes to easing the pain and stiffness that OA imposes. So I want you to add extra daily servings of these foods, and I want you to be extra stringent about avoiding certain foods that aren't on the plan. You'll probably see that within a month or two (sorry, there's no overnight fix for OA pain) your pain will ease and your joints will be moving smoothly and more comfortably.

Eat these foods more often:

- Wild Alaskan salmon and other cold-water fish, especially sardines
- Freshly ground flaxseed (add to smoothies and salads)
- Organic, omega-3-fortified eggs
- Avocados
- Walnuts
- Tart cherries, blueberries, and other low-sugar berries (off season, you can often find frozen organic berries at your supermarket)
- Garlic, onions, and scallions

Just Say No to Dairy

Arthritis is a perfect illustration of why dairy foods are crossed off the No More Pills Plan. Over the years, I've observed that in almost every family where osteoarthritis supposedly "runs in the family," reactivity to dairy also "runs in the family." I've had many patients whose arthritic pain literally disappeared when they got off dairy, so in my experience, it's well worth a trial if you have arthritic pain.

I remember clearly, even though it was years ago, a patient whom I will call Tricia C., who came to see me in the late '80s. Tricia was in her midfifties and had arthritic pain in her hands. She even had some swelling in her finger joints that looked like the kind that doesn't go away. I suspected that she was reactive to dairy.

She went on a dairy-free diet and came weekly for a series of 10 acupuncture treatments. Her hand pain went away, and what was even more amazing to me (and to her) was that the swelling in her joints near the ends of her fingers reduced. I had learned in medical school that this kind of arthritic swelling was progressive and not reversible, but I saw something different with my own eyes, and I started to act on it.

At around the same time, my dad started to complain that he was having trouble with his fingers, too. He had pain, and he also had swelling, including little, hard bony nodules on top of the joint called Heberden's nodes. These were thought to be irreversible, and if they caused him trouble, the only known option was to have them surgically removed. He lived 3 hours away, so it was impossible for me to give him weekly acupuncture treatments. But he was someone who would follow my instructions to a T and was willing to commit to a daily program, so I gave him a set of acupressure points to press on while he watched TV. He followed through diligently, and wonder of wonders, his nodules went away. I also asked him to cut back on his dairy, too—a tough proposition, since he was raised on an Iowa farm! He was in his seventies back then, and his hand problems went away until the age of 86, when he developed a heart valve infection. And he played tennis until he was 84!

Avoid these totally:

- Polyunsaturated vegetable oils, such as corn and soy
- Partially hydrogenated oils (aka trans fats) found in processed foods
- Processed foods containing artificial coloring and chemical preservatives

Get Right with Spice

Your spice rack contains a few bottles that vie with pills for their ability to ease OA pain. Two important facts about using spices to augment OA treatments: First, unlike NSAIDs, spices rarely have side effects; NSAIDs increase your risk for heart attack and stroke, plus they can also cause stomach and intestinal bleeding. Second, spices don't work as quickly as drugs do, so you have to use them regularly and frequently—or, better still, use them in cooking as well as in supplement form (see page 136).

These three spices top my list for helping ease arthritis.

Turmeric (*Curcuma longa*). This spice is related to ginger; its most medically active compound is curcumin. This spice that gives curry, ballpark mustard, and bread-and-butter pickles their brilliant golden hue comes from the plant's rhizome (its underground stem connected to the roots). Curcumin is a compound that researchers have been feverishly studying for many years. It has a number of medicinal effects, not the least of which is its ability to chill inflammation. You can use this exotically tangy spice to enhance your cooking. It adds a distinctive touch to scrambled eggs and curries, and it's a wonderful partner for butternut and other winter squash dishes. Just make sure the food you're adding it to contains a little fat to help your body absorb the curcumin.

Ginger (*Zingiber officinale*). If you ask me, ginger's got it all. Its spicy, warming flavor gives a nice zing (maybe that's where its scientific name originated?) to foods both sweet and savory—think smoothies, soups, stews, roasts, salad dressings, fish, vegetables, and even the occasional dessert. Ginger enhances most foods you add it to. Beyond its flavor, ginger is a medicine, one that the Chinese have been using at least since 3000 BC. Among its many medicinally active compounds, the diarylheptanoids (curcumin also contains these)[10, 11] may reduce inflammation and arthritis pain as well as help block the release of inflammatory substances such as prostaglandins.[12, 13]

Black pepper (*Piper nigrum*). You probably never thought of plain old black pepper as a healing spice, but in fact, it's a common remedy in traditional Chinese medicine. Pepper is packed with compounds that have many healthful actions—including anti-inflammatory properties. In a 2013 test-tube study, researchers looked at the effects of piperine, an active pepper constituent. They pretreated human OA chondrocytes (cartilage cells) with black pepper and then zapped the cells with an inflammatory protein. Through some very fancy and nearly incomprehensible (unless you're an immunology researcher) science, they learned that piperine actually inhibited the cells' inflammatory activity, leading the researchers to conclude that piperine could be an effective OA treatment. To be sure, my suggestion that you spice things up with black pepper is certainly a long way from what these researchers found in the lab. However, as a physician who's studied Chinese herbal medicine, I'm very aware of black pepper's role in dampening pain and reducing inflammation, so I encourage you to increase your use of this tasty spice. One more word of advice: Do use a pepper mill to grind peppercorns freshly for each use.[14]

Add Some Acupuncture

I've been trained in acupuncture and been using it for decades in my practice, where I've seen it benefit any number of conditions. It's been frequently studied and proved to be successful time and time again for arthritis pain and other conditions. One study I found interesting was reported in the *Journal of the American Geriatrics Society* in 2010. In the study, the researchers tested acupuncture on people suffering from painful knee OA who also had trouble sleeping. Since pain often interrupts sleep—which, in a vicious cycle, causes more pain—the researchers were hoping to see whether acupuncture could, in a sense, kill two birds with one stone. And in fact, that's just what happened. Acupuncture improved sleep disturbances and helped ease pain.

These days, many insurance policies cover acupuncture treatments. To find a licensed, qualified practitioner, visit nccaom.org.

Be Smart about Supplements

I frequently recommend dietary supplements to my patients who have osteoarthritis. I consider some of these to be an essential part of everyone's OA treatment plan. Others work better for some people, depending on their individual conditions. Here are the supplements I use and why.

Fish oil/omega-3 fatty acids. If you think of your arthritic joints as squeaky hinges that quiet when you oil them, you can see how "lubricating" your joints by taking fish oil might be a helpful solution. Beyond the too-easy metaphor, however, is scientific evidence that the right kind of fish oil supplement, at the correct dose, can help ease OA pain because of its ability to decrease inflammation.

Dose: NOW Foods Ultra Omega-3, 1 capsule a day.[15, 16]

Glucosamine/chondroitin. Studies have delivered slightly inscrutable results on this combination of naturally occurring substances. But many people find the combo useful for helping ease their arthritis pain, and the good news is that some studies show that it can actually help rebuild cartilage. You have to take this supplement for at least 2 to 4 months before experiencing improvement, though some people do feel better sooner.

Dose: 1.5 grams a day, taken once or in three 500-milligram doses.[17, 18]

Curcumin. I mentioned turmeric as a spice to regularly add to your food for its anti-inflammatory benefits. In addition, consider taking it in supplement form. In a recent study, taking curcumin was as effective for pain relief as taking ibuprofen but caused less abdominal distress.

Dose: Two 500-milligram capsules a day. It may be better absorbed when taken with a meal containing some fat and a dash or two of black pepper.[19]

SAMe (S-adenosylmethionine). This is a compound found naturally in every cell of the body. It's key to your body's production of the neurotransmitters dopamine and serotonin as well as cartilage components. In studies, SAMe has proven effective for OA and joint pain and stiffness, and several studies show that its benefits last longer and that it has fewer side effects than NSAIDs.[20] In one 8-week-long 2009 study, 134 patients were randomly assigned to one of two groups: One group got 400 milligrams of SAMe three times a day; the other group got 1,000 milligrams of nabumetone, an NSAID, once a day. At the end of the study, patients rated the SAMe as equally effective as the NSAID for pain treatment.[21]

Get Moving, Slowly but Surely

"Use it or lose it" is a great reminder about getting up and walking, especially when you have OA. Sure, the pain can be enough to keep you nailed to your La-Z-Boy watching *Law & Order* reruns, but I can tell you that that's absolutely the worst thing you can do for yourself. We know that physical activity is proven to ease OA symptoms. I don't want you to feel that you have to become a gym rat, but I do want you up and moving rather than spending hours at a time sitting. See Chapter 4 for some easy walking and yoga programs. In particular, stretching is excellent for helping ease arthritis pain, especially if you've been inactive for a while. Your gym or Y might have a special class specifically for people with OA—many even have pool programs, which combine the warmth of the pool water with gentle exercises that put no pressure on your joints.

Try Some EFT

You might not think about pain as a stressor, but it's one of the most significant stressors the body can face. Many people have found the emotional freedom technique, covered in Chapter 5, to be a quick and effective way to deal with the chronic pain of arthritis. See page 106 to get started.

• •

DR. HOWARD'S Q&A

Q. I have knee pain that my doctor confirms is due to osteoarthritis. Besides diet, what's the one thing I can take or do to ease the pain so I don't have to slow my walking program?

A. You may want to stop your walking program and start a water exercise program instead. Water exercise has actually been proven to help arthritis; you can often find classes at Ys and community centers. Also, a qualified traditional Chinese medicine practitioner can give you Chinese herbal formulas to help with the inflammation and pain, as well as acupuncture—both of these, in my experience, are extremely helpful.

Cardiovascular Disease

Cardiovascular disease refers to disease that affects the heart and blood vessels. Since the heart is the main "pump" that circulates blood throughout your body and the blood vessels are the "pipes" that carry oxygen and other nutrients to every cell, tissue, and organ in your body, when your heart or blood vessels are in trouble, so are you.

Though your genes and your family history can influence whether or not you become a candidate for disease, your lifestyle is a far more significant factor. One thing I know for certain: The No More Pills Plan is the first line of defense against heart disease, and it can improve the condition at every stage of its development. The end results of following my plan could be that you (a) could prevent cardiovascular disease, (b) might be able to reduce your pills, or (c) could stop taking some of your pills. The answer depends on your personal health factors and how closely you follow the plan.

Cardiovascular disease also refers to the several intertwined problems that lead to one in four deaths in America every year. Underpinning these problems, quite often, is a condition called atherosclerosis (hardening of the arteries), which develops when a sticky substance called plaque builds up on artery walls. Plaque buildup narrows and stiffens the arteries, restricting bloodflow. Plaques that rupture and break away from artery walls become blood clots that can stop bloodflow and cause heart attacks when they form in the heart's blood vessels or strokes when they form in the brain's blood vessels.[1, 2] (Arteriosclerosis is another condition involving stiffening of the arteries that doesn't involve plaque buildup.)

High cholesterol contributes to the buildup of atherosclerotic deposits on artery walls. Another major problem under the umbrella of cardiovascular disease is high blood pressure.

Wind Down High Blood Pressure

High blood pressure is called a silent killer because this central component of heart disease causes no outward symptoms; your first indication of a problem is likely to be when your doctor straps the cuff around your arm and delivers the unwelcome news.

Blood pressure numbers are a measurement of the force of the blood that pushes against artery walls as your heart pumps. If your blood pressure remains high over time (a condition called hypertension), it damages your heart, your arteries, and other organs. One in three Americans has hypertension (HTN). Blood pressure is measured in two numbers: systolic (the first number) and diastolic (the second). In a normal blood pressure reading, numbers should be less than 120/80. People are considered to have prehypertension when pressure reads 120 to 139/80 to 89. Physicians diagnose stage 1 hypertension at 140 to 159/90 to 99; stage 2 is 160 or higher over 100 or higher.

But blood pressure isn't static. It's lower when you're asleep or in a deeply relaxed state—when you're meditating, for example. It rises when you're awake, active, excited, or nervous.[4] That's why it's so important to spend periods of time in a relaxed state as often as possible. It gives your cardiovascular system a much-needed rest and allows your circulation to flow freely. The following steps (along with the other suggestions in this section) can help prevent you from having to take pills to lower your blood pressure.

Master a form of meditation. Researchers who searched medical studies for evidence about meditation's effects on heart disease and blood pressure discovered that several forms of meditation had positive effects. They learned that mindfulness-based stress reduction, transcendental meditation, progressive muscle relaxation, and stress management courses effectively help lower blood pressure.[5]

Try chair massage. If you think that massage is a luxurious indulgence reserved for special treats, think again. Even a 10- to 15-minute chair massage helps lower high blood pressure or prehypertension. Here's the science: Iranian researchers studied the effect of massage on 50 women with prehypertension. Twenty-five of the women got 10 to 15 minutes of Swedish massage three times a week for 10 sessions; the other 25 spent the same amount of time relaxing. After the 10 sessions, the systolic blood pressure of the women in the massage group dropped from a mean of 128 to 116. The BP of the control group went up about a point. The results persisted at least 3 days following the last massage. What's nice about this study is that it shows even a few chair massage sessions can work wonders to lower blood pressure. Results of this study were published in 2013 in the *International Journal of Preventive Medicine*. Other studies have confirmed massage's positive impact on lowering blood pressure.[6, 7]

Gobble up blueberries. Eating just one serving of yummy blueberries a week can drop your risks of having high blood pressure by 10 percent, according to research published in the *American Journal of Clinical Nutrition* in 2011. Blueberries are loaded with powerful antioxidants known as anthocyanins. This compound also occurs in strawberries and raspberries, so be sure to enjoy these sweet treats, too.[8]

Take probiotics. In their 2014 study released by the American Heart Association, Australian researchers examined nine high-quality studies involving more than 500 people that measured the effects of taking probiotics on high blood pressure. They concluded that taking probiotics can lower blood pressure. I recommend Renew Life Ultimate Flora capsules that contain either 30 billion or 50 billion of these good bacteria. Generally, the older you get, the more probiotics you need.[9]

Put two dates on your calendar. People with high blood pressure who check in with their doctors twice a year are three times more likely to keep blood pressure under control than people who visit less frequently, according to a 2014 study from the University of South Carolina School of Medicine, published in the journal *Circulation*.[10]

Could It Be My Pills?

Prescription, over-the-counter, and recreational drugs can cause high blood pressure.[11] Among them:

Amphetamines, ecstasy, and cocaine

Corticosteroids

Cyclosporine

Erythropoietin

Estrogens (including birth control pills) and other hormones

Migraine medications

Nasal decongestants

Cough/cold and antiasthma medications

Drinking alcoholic beverages can also increase blood pressure.

The Truth about High Cholesterol

Quick: Define cholesterol. If you say it's a fat in your bloodstream that most people have too much of, it might surprise you to learn that you're only partially right. Actually, cholesterol is the most common steroid found in the human body. It has two key roles: to help the body produce such life-sustaining compounds as vitamin D, progesterone, estrogen, and other hormones and to help cells absorb nutrients and release waste products. When levels of certain kinds of cholesterol—low-density lipoprotein (LDL) and triglycerides—are too high, cholesterol can build up in your artery's walls, reducing bloodflow and setting the stage for heart attacks and strokes.

Up until recently, we've believed that lowering our blood levels of cholesterol via low-fat diets would keep our hearts healthy. This mistaken notion triggered food companies to pump out tons of low-fat and fat-free processed foods that were laced with salt, sugar, and, often, heavily processed grains to compensate for the lack of flavor and mouthfeel that fat delivers. As a result, Americans actually became more obese—and less healthy. We discovered that diets rich in omega-3 fats, such as the Mediterranean diet and the Paleo diet (the No More Pills Plan combines aspects of both of these plans), are far better ways to keep cholesterol levels within a healthy range.[12, 13]

In 2013, the American Heart Association and the American College of Cardiology did something that many medical experts, including me, found shocking: They issued new cholesterol guidelines that suggested that millions of otherwise healthy Americans should start taking statin drugs to lower their cholesterol. Two eminent physicians, John D. Abramson, MD, on the faculty of Harvard Medical School, and Rita F. Redberg, MD, a cardiologist at the University of California, San Francisco Medical Center and the editor of *JAMA Internal Medicine*, took issue with those guidelines in a *New York Times* editorial in November 2013.

Here's what they said: "This announcement is not the result of a sudden epidemic of heart disease, nor is it based on new data showing the benefits of lower cholesterol. Instead, it is a consequence of simply expanding the definition of who should take the drugs—a decision that will benefit the pharmaceutical industry more than anyone else."[14]

My opinion? I think statins are the perfect example of how the pharmaceutical industry twists the truth and strong-arms the medical community (and patients) into believing something that isn't actually true. To understand what I mean, you have to understand the medical research term *number needed to treat*. This refers to the number of people who have to take a drug for a single person to benefit from it.

For statins, the number needed to treat is huge. In a 2011 review of statin research, the study author reported that when it comes to statins, *1,000 people would need to be treated for 1 year to prevent one heart disease- related death*. That means many people would have to cope with statins' side effects (not to mention, they would also have to shell out for the cost of the drugs) to prevent the death of one person from heart disease.[15]

Interestingly, researchers who conducted a gigantic 2013 *BMJ* analysis of studies comparing drug treatment for heart disease to exercise (see page

150) pointed out that our National Cholesterol Education Program (NCEP) used to advise taking statins only after lifestyle changes had failed. Then, noted the researchers, we changed the program guidelines—we lowered the threshold for drug treatment, which meant that doctors were encouraged to prescribe statins to more people than ever.[16]

My bottom line: I believe that this is terrible math and that using statins to lower heart disease risk—especially as a primary treatment—is simply terrible medicine.

Furthermore, I believe that the best way to achieve these numbers is not by popping a pill but by following the delectable No More Pills Plan, which is rich in the kind of healthy fats and foods that help lower cholesterol. These tips can help, too.

The Statin-Cataract Connection

According to two new studies, using statins can significantly boost the risk of developing cataracts severe enough to require surgery, said Canadian researchers from the University of British Columbia in Vancouver in late 2014.[17]

Crunch on walnuts. Adding about 1½ ounces of walnuts a day to your diet can lower "bad" cholesterol by about 10 mg/dL, which is a significant reduction, according to a 2014 study published in the journal *Metabolism*.[18]

Sip some red wine. Drinking a few glasses of red wine a week is a relaxing strategy I particularly love—and it helps lower cholesterol. "Antioxidants contained in red wines such as Cabernet Sauvignon, Merlot, and Pinot Noir help slow down the oxidation of HDL and LDL cholesterol," says Vincent Rifici, PhD, of the Robert Wood Johnson Medical School in New Brunswick, New Jersey.[19]

Take a nightly stroll. A nice 30-minute walk at any time of the day, done regularly at least 5 days a week, will help lower your cholesterol. But strolling after dinner offers even better benefits, according to a 2014 Chinese study of 330 people. The study revealed that taking an evening walk drops cholesterol numbers a bit lower than a morning walk does.[20]

Consider red yeast rice (RYR). This natural supplement, long used in traditional Chinese medicine, is made by culturing rice with a strain of yeast. It's chemically similar to statin drugs, though at weaker concentrations. "I recommend RYR to people who haven't had a bypass, stent, or previous heart attack and for people who'd rather not take statins for high cholesterol," says David Becker, MD, a cardiologist in Philadelphia who has published several RYR studies. Most people with moderately high cholesterol do benefit from RYR, but it may not be strong enough for people with cholesterol higher than 190 mg/dL, says Dr. Becker.[21] I like NOW Foods RYR. Start with 600 milligrams.

Raise Levels of This Cholesterol

One type of cholesterol, HDL (high-density lipoprotein), is healthy for your heart, so you want to raise your HDL number if it's too low. Ideally, your HDL levels should be above 60; if they're below 40, you need to take action. Here's how.

Pick up policosanol. This sugarcane compound is proven to safely lower "bad" cholesterol and can raise HDL cholesterol by a healthy 17 percent, according to one study.[22] In a study of 437 patients, those who took policosanol experienced a 28 percent increase in HDL cholesterol. You can find this supplement at most drugstores.

Cholesterol by the Numbers

Here's what your cholesterol numbers should be, as far as I'm concerned. I use the older guidelines because the new ones have yet to be proven. Like many other doctors, I believe that the new guidelines, which lowered the cholesterol treatment threshold, were put in place simply to sell statins.[23, 24, 25]

Total cholesterol:	Less than 200 mg/dL
LDL (bad) cholesterol:	Less than 130 mg/dL
HDL (good) cholesterol:	Above 40 mg/dL for men, 50 mg/dL for women
Triglycerides:	Less than 150 mg/dL

Consider niacin. The National Cholesterol Education Program considers niacin (vitamin B_3) as a top choice for normalizing blood lipid levels. Studies show that it raises HDL levels by up to 40 percent, while it reduces total cholesterol 10 to 25 percent and triglycerides by a whopping 50 percent.[26] Choose the form called no-flush niacin. *Note:* Do not take niacin if you are taking Lipitor or another lipid-lowering drug.

The No More Pills Plan Helps Beat Heart Disease

Hundreds of studies confirm the benefits of diets similar to the No More Pills Plan for beating all the components of heart disease. There are so many studies that listing them would take more space than I have! In fact, researchers began linking diet with heart disease as far back as 1935. And now we even have proof that the right diet can equal the benefits of certain pills for lowering heart disease risks—without pills' side effects.

For example, in one landmark study published in the *Journal of the American Medical Association* back in 2003, researchers proved that a diet rich in fruits, vegetables, and nuts delivered about the same results as did a common statin drug. The diet was as effective as the drug for lowering C-reactive protein (an inflammation marker implicated in raising heart disease risk) and heart-unhealthy LDL cholesterol by about 30 percent.[27]

What's more, it doesn't take long for a heart-healthy diet like the No More Pills Plan to improve heart health. In just 3 months, eating a Mediterranean-style diet similar to this plan reduced the risk of heart disease by 15 percent, when compared to a low-fat diet, according to a 2005 study published in the *American Journal of Clinical Nutrition.*[28]

"It's never too late," says Bonnie Spring, PhD, professor in preventive medicine at Northwestern University Feinberg School of Medicine in Chicago.[29] Dr. Spring and her team recently studied data from 5,000 participants in a lifestyle study and learned that by adopting healthy lifestyle strategies—such as maintaining a healthy weight, eating a healthy diet, being physically active, and not smoking—people could improve the health of their coronary arteries.

According to Dr. Spring, her team's discoveries helped debunk two myths held by some health care professionals: One, that it's nearly impossible to change a patient's behavior. (About 25 percent of the people in her study made changes on their own.) And two, that once damage has been done to coronary arteries, it's irreversible. It turns out that you can reverse the damage. Though the people in her study were young adults, Dr. Spring says that reversing heart disease is possible at any age; it just takes a commitment to making a lifestyle change, which is what the No More Pills Plan is all about.[30]

What is it about the No More Pills Plan that's specifically helpful for heart disease? Simple, really. It's high in fiber, low in sodium (none of those sodium-bomb processed foods, for example), and loaded with fruits, vegetables, and good fats. A diet like this is one of the healthy habits that can control and potentially even reverse the natural progression of coronary artery disease, according to a 2014 study published in the journal *Circulation*.

Top Foods for the Healthiest Heart

One trick to creating a diet your heart will love is to keep it varied, says Arthur Agatston, MD, the renowned cardiologist who created the South Beach Diet. Eating many different types of organic, rainbow-colored fruits and vegetables, eggs, wild fish, and grass-fed meats means you'll get the widest possible assortment of heart-healthy phytochemicals, antioxidants, and good fats. But even among those great choices, some foods give your heart an even healthier edge, like these:

Wild salmon. This succulent powerhouse fish is rich in omega-3s and the potent antioxidant selenium, which studies show protects the heart.

Extra virgin olive oil. Swap this beautiful oil for less healthful vegetable oils; it contains higher levels of good fats and antioxidants to help unclog your arteries. Another good fat choice, though pricey, is avocado oil, which in a 2005 study proved to help decrease hardening of the arteries.[31]

Walnuts and almonds. Again, it's the omega-3s that make these nuts such wonderfully powerful heart foods; both are great sources of fiber.

Brussels sprouts, broccoli, and cauliflower. These cruciferous veggies reduce inflammation in the cardiovascular system and improve the health of your blood vessels.

Spinach and asparagus. Both of these are rich in the B vitamin folate, which lowers homocysteine levels. Homocysteine is an amino acid that plays a role in heart disease, stroke, and peripheral artery disease. Up to half of all people with heart disease have high homocysteine levels, compared with just 5 percent of healthy people. High homocysteine levels are implicated in severe atherosclerosis. What's more, it is suspected that homocysteine promotes vascular problems by damaging blood vessel linings and enabling blood clot formation.[32]

Garlic. Cooking with garlic reduces heart attack risk in three ways: It makes red blood cells less sticky, thus reducing blood clot risk; it prevents damage to arteries; and it discourages cholesterol from lining those arteries and making them so narrow that blockages are likely.[33] But here's a trick: First, make sure to chop, slice, or mash it, because doing so combines two garlic compounds into the potent allicin, which is responsible for garlic's health benefits. Then, let it sit for 10 minutes. Add the garlic close to the end of the cooking time to preserve its power.[34]

Chia seeds. Emerging research points to chia seeds' ability to lower cholesterol, triglycerides, and blood pressure, according to the Academy of Nutrition and Dietetics.[35]

Blueberries and strawberries. Eating three or more half-cup servings of blueberries or strawberries a week can lower your heart attack risk by 34 percent, according to a 2013 Harvard School of Public Health study that reviewed data from more than 90,000 women over 18 years.[36]

Apples. Rich in polyphenols, which protect cells from free-radical damage, these crunchy fruits also contain pectin and fiber, which block cholesterol absorption and help clear it from the bloodstream. And they just may, as the old saying goes, keep the doctor away! Tips: Vary the kinds of apples you enjoy and leave the peels on—they contain most of the fruits' antioxidants.

Avocados. They are laced with monounsaturated fats, the good fats that help lower cholesterol and reduce the risk of blood clots. And try avocado oil, which can help modify fatty acids in the tissues that surround the heart.[37, 38]

Don't Eat These: Scratch Killer Fats Off Your Menu

Trans fats are among the unhealthiest fake food ingredients ever created. The food industry concocted trans fats years ago via a process that adds hydrogen to liquid vegetable oils to create a solid fat. They're cheap and easy for processors to use, and they give processed foods a taste and mouth-feel designed to make them addictive. On food labels, these killers are listed as "partially hydrogenated fats."

Trans fats raise levels of unhealthy LDL cholesterol and lower levels of healthy HDL cholesterol. The American Heart Association says that trans fats boost your risks for heart attacks and strokes.

The good news is, if you stick to the No More Pills Plan, you won't be eating trans fats, except for the tiny amount that naturally occurs in grass-fed, organic meats. What's more, the addition of trans fats to foods has become less frequent since the FDA took away their "generally recognized as safe" designation in 2013. Still, they haven't disappeared entirely, so read labels carefully. And keep this in mind: The ability of your cells to absorb nutrients and eliminate wastes depends on the quality of the fats in their membranes. Those yucky trans fats stick around (pun intended) for *120 days*. That's 4 months! What do you want your cells to have: nice clear fats like organic olive oil or fake trans fats, which are gunky oils that corrode the health of your blood vessels?[39]

Healthy Heart Supplements

I often recommend these six key supplements to patients. In studies—and in my experience—they have been found to help guard against heart disease.

Take some fish oil. The two omega-3 fatty acids found in fish oil, eicosapentaenoic and docosahexaenoic acids (EPA and DHA for short), have an impressive body of research proving their therapeutic role in protecting the health of your heart. I like NOW Foods Ultra Omega-3. Take one a day.

Get your fill of folate. Folate (vitamin B_9) is a key heart-health nutrient. As mentioned earlier, folate (along with B_6 and B_{12}) helps lower high levels of homocysteine, an amino acid that promotes blood vessel problems. (Folic acid is its synthetic form.) Women who get at least 400 micrograms of folate a day have a 20 to 30 percent lower risk for heart disease, according to studies.[40]

Protect your D levels. A study presented at a 2014 meeting of the European Society of Cardiology showed that vitamin D deficiencies worsen brain function following a heart attack—and lead to a sharply higher risk of death following a sudden heart attack. In the study of 53 patients, three

Turn That Frown Upside Down

A 2014 study confirms that stress, hostility, and depression play as big a role in your cardiovascular health as do your cholesterol levels, blood pressure, and even whether or not you smoke tobacco, says Susan Everson-Rose, PhD, lead study author and associate professor of medicine at the University of Minnesota in Minneapolis. In her study of more than 6,700 adults, ages 45 to 84, she learned that those with the highest levels of stress, depression, and hostility were sharply more likely to have a stroke or transient ischemic attack (TIA) than happier, less stressed people.

Compared to people with low stress, low depression, and low anger scores, those with the highest scores for these states of mind were:

- 86 percent more likely to have a stroke or TIA for high depressive scores

- 59 percent more likely to have a stroke or TIA for the highest chronic stress scores

- More than twice as likely to have a stroke or TIA for the highest hostility scores[41]

Many strategies in this book can help you combat depression, stress, and hostility. Cognitive behavioral therapy is a good place to start.

I often refer people who deal with crazy-making amounts of stress to the works of my pal Loretta LaRoche. She wrote the book *Life Is Not a Stress Rehearsal.* It's funny and irreverent and a great way to gently jolt you into a healthier frame of mind. To learn more, visit lorettalaroche.com.

times as many patients with vitamin D deficiencies had poor brain function 6 months after their attack as did people with normal D levels. What's more, nearly one-third of the people with low D levels died within 6 months after their heart attacks, compared to none of the patients with normal D levels. I recommend at least 1,000 IU of vitamin D[42] for most adults, but keep in mind that a recent study showed that at least 50 percent of adults over the age of 60 need 2,000 IU a day. That's five times the minimum daily requirement of vitamin D, which is still 400 IU, though many of us hope for this number to be raised.

Add CoQ10. This antioxidant is a must, especially if you're taking statin drugs. One potential cause of the muscle pain that is a known side effect of statins is the fact that these drugs deplete blood levels of CoQ10. Take 100 milligrams a day.[43]

Take AGE (aged garlic extract). If you're not eating garlic regularly (you should be!), consider taking an aged garlic extract supplement to reduce your risk of developing blood clots and to keep arteries healthy. Take 600 milligrams twice a day.[44]

Mine some magnesium. Magnesium plays a role in keeping blood pressure stable. If you have low blood levels of magnesium (ask your doctor to check), taking 400 milligrams of magnesium every evening can help.[45] *Note:* It's best to take minerals, especially calcium and magnesium, at night.

Exercise Beats Pills for Heart Disease

You know that your heart is a muscle. Like other muscles in the body, when you don't exercise it, it gets flabby. And a flabby heart does your vigor and longevity absolutely no favors whatsoever.

If you're not a fan of taking pills, you'll be especially interested in the results of a recent review of more than 57 clinical trials that focused on exercise; it included nearly 15,000 people. The study was published in the renowned journal *BMJ* in 2013.

What did this study reveal? Exercise is about as effective as some heart drugs (statins, beta-blockers, antiplatelet drugs, and ACE inhibitors) for preventing heart disease deaths. Here's what the researchers said: "Exercise and many drug interventions are often potentially similar in terms of their mortality benefits." They concluded that exercise should be considered as an alternative to—or at least recommended alongside—drug therapy. But the sad truth is that only about 33 percent of primary care doctors prescribe the "exercise pill."[46]

If you really want to do your heart some good and lessen your chances for having to take drugs (or potentially be able to reduce the amount you take, or even stop taking them, under your doctor's supervision), please follow the walking program with interval training on page 75. Aerobic interval exercise has been proven to improve heart health in people with coronary artery disease. Just make sure you are "cleared" for exercise by your doctor before you start your program.[47]

● ●

DR. HOWARD'S Q&A

Q. I have a family history of heart disease, so I'm extra careful to eat healthfully, stick to my recommended weight, and walk nearly every day. I just turned 62. Should I start seeing a cardiologist in addition to my family doctor, just in case?

A. Absolutely! Because of your family history, ask your primary care doctor for a referral to a cardiologist and make an appointment for a consultation.

Chronic Fatigue Syndrome and Fibromyalgia

Chronic fatigue syndrome is a poorly understood chronic condition that can leave you feeling too exhausted to get through the tasks of your day. But it's not just a feeling; it's a very real, very burdensome illness. This section will discuss this chronic condition, along with another often-related condition: fibromyalgia.

Chronic Fatigue Syndrome

Fatigue, even bone-melting exhaustion, occasionally comes with the territory of 21st-century life. You may be a breadwinner or a co-breadwinner with a demanding job, and on top of that, a mother (today, 20-something kids demand almost as much energy as the young ones do), a supportive spouse, a daughter of aging parents, or the go-to pal for close friends. You may feel as if you're the tent pole that holds your extended family together. It's no wonder you're exhausted from time to time.

But when your exhaustion lasts longer than 6 consecutive months and interferes with your daily activities, and you've enlisted your doctor's diagnostic skills and still can't connect your fatigue to a medical condition, you could have the debilitating condition known by two names: chronic fatigue syndrome (CFS) or chronic fatigue immune dysfunction syndrome (CFIDS). In the United Kingdom, it's myalgic encephalomyelitis/chronic fatigue syndrome. If you've got it, you don't much care what it's called; you just want to get rid of it and get your life back.

Its symptoms include:

- Severe, chronic fatigue that lasts longer than 6 months (when all other medical causes have been excluded)

Plus, along with the fatigue, four or more of these symptoms:[1]

- Exhaustion lasting more than 24 hours following exertion
- Unrefreshing sleep

It's Not All in Your Head

No test exists to prove whether or not you have chronic fatigue syndrome (CFS). Not so long ago, if your doctor couldn't diagnose your symptoms, she might have suggested they were psychosomatic—that is, all in your head. Try telling that to acclaimed author Laura Hillenbrand, who wrote the bestselling book *Seabiscuit* back in 2001 while coping with extreme CFS symptoms. Hillenbrand, now 34, can barely enjoy the fruits of her runaway success. She deals with night sweats, fevers, and extreme exhaustion, and for days at a time, she can't leave her home in Washington, DC. Though, as of this writing, no treatment has proved effective for Hillenbrand, she says that "writing this book was a matter of dignifying my place in this world. I wasn't going to let CFS defeat me."[2]

Fortunately, most people with CFS have milder symptoms. Still, you may have good days and bad days; symptoms can swing from mild to severe from morning to evening for no apparent reason. And I believe that the No More Pills Plan can help many people, even those with severe symptoms like Hillenbrand's.

Commonly, CFS can overcome a previously fit and active person following an infection of some kind (Hillenbrand's started with a bad case of food poisoning). Less common triggers include exposure to toxins or pesticides, a major trauma or stress (a bad accident, for example), surgical procedures, and even pregnancy. And sometimes you can't pinpoint a cause: Your energy just starts flagging, and you begin feeling lousy and ill and no one knows why.

Experts have no idea what causes CFS. I believe it's a complex collection of triggers, many of which most physicians don't even consider when they evaluate your symptoms. Some experts link CFS to the Epstein-Barr virus or cytomegalovirus, but viral links certainly aren't apparent in all people with CFS.

- Substantially impaired concentration or short-term memory
- Muscle pain
- Pain in multiple joints without swelling or redness
- Headaches of new type, pattern, or severity
- Tender lymph nodes
- Frequent or recurring sore throat

These symptoms must have occurred at the same time, not before, the fatigue began. Symptoms must have persisted or recurred during the 6 months of illness.

Having come this far in this book, you probably know where I'm going with this: When it comes to a somewhat murky diagnosis such as CFS, let's first look to your diet and see if you're reactive to any of the foods you're eating. You could also be deficient in key vitamins and minerals. The last thing I'd want to do as a first-line treatment is to prescribe pills, such as antidepressants or sleeping pills, which are common CFS treatments.[3]

In general, my approach for treating CFS will be similar to my treatment program for a kindred condition, fibromyalgia.

Fibromyalgia

If having chronic fatigue syndrome makes you exhausted, fibromyalgia makes you hurt. It's a chronic pain syndrome whose additional symptoms include fatigue and specific body points that are tender to the touch. In my experience, people can have symptoms of both CFS and fibromyalgia.

The latest common thinking on fibromyalgia is that it may have a genetic component and that stress plays a role: It often surfaces after you've experienced significantly stressful events—emotional, medical, or physical.[4]

I call both fibromyalgia and CFS wastebasket diagnoses—terms that physicians use instead of considering all of the other potential factors for your problem, including hormone imbalances, vitamin and mineral deficiencies, and undiagnosed food allergies. I also believe, frankly, that the number of fibromyalgia diagnoses is on the rise thanks to the major marketing campaign by the makers of the widely promoted fibromyalgia drug pregabalin (Lyrica). Unfortunately, this drug doesn't come without the potential for some negative side effects (see "Pregabalin Side Effects").

Pregabalin Side Effects

This antiseizure medication might be the first thing that comes to your doctor's mind when she's weighing treatments for your fibromyalgia. But this pill comes with the potential for disturbing and dangerous side effects.[5, 6]

10 percent of people experience:
- Dizziness or drowsiness

1 to 10 percent of people experience:
- Visual problems
- Lack of coordination of muscle movements
- Memory problems
- Speech problems
- Constipation
- Dry mouth

- Loss of sex drive/erectile dysfunction
- Weight gain

Rare:
- Serious, even life-threatening, allergic reactions
- Suicidal thoughts or actions
- Swelling of hands, legs, and feet

If the side effects of a drug like pregabalin (FYI, the antidepressants often prescribed for fibromyalgia and CFS have similar side effects) don't convince you to try safer, nondrug therapies, maybe the math will. Turns out, the odds that a drug such as pregabalin or an antidepressant will ease your symptoms are pretty low, says Winfried Häuser, MD, associate professor of psychosomatic medicine at the Klinikum Saarbrücken in Saarbrücken, Germany. Dr. Häuser is a world-renowned fibromyalgia researcher and expert.[7]

According to Dr. Häuser, out of every four to six people who take an antidepressant or pregabalin for fibromyalgia, one person will experience about one-third less pain. "No drug is very good when it comes to easing any kind of chronic pain condition," says Dr. Häuser. However, there is good news:

Two therapies offer sustained relief for fibromyalgia—and are better than drugs, he notes. Aerobic exercise and cognitive behavioral therapies are scientifically proven as effective fibromyalgia treatments and are safe, says Dr. Häuser.[8]

The No More Pills Plan for Fibromyalgia and CFS

I begin my treatment of both fibromyalgia and CFS (since some people have symptoms that are common to both conditions) by addressing my patients' diets. First, I make sure that no undiagnosed food allergies are present that could be causing the symptoms.

Then I help my patient transition to the No More Pills Plan, adapting it as necessary, depending on the results of her allergy tests. In the beginning stages of treatment, it's critical to follow the diet strictly to best ease the exhaustion and pain.

A huge benefit of the No More Pills Plan for people with chronic fatigue syndrome and fibromyalgia is that it's rich in antioxidants. These are particularly important for fighting both conditions, because neutralizing free radicals, the job antioxidants perform, helps prevent cell damage that can contribute to the exhaustion and pain caused by CFS and fibromyalgia.

Make sure to add these super antioxidants to your daily diet. All must be organic.

- Green, black, hibiscus, and rooibos teas
- Berries of all colors—blueberries, raspberries, strawberries, blackberries
- Red, purple, and blue grapes
- Dark green veggies[9]

Note: The No More Pills Plan is about as clean a diet as I can devise. That means it doesn't contain processed foods, nonorganic meat or produce, or junk or fast foods. For most people, an occasional treat such as a fast-food meal or a pizza, for example, won't be a problem. But even one such diet departure could worsen symptoms of fibromyalgia and CFS. People who have one of these conditions may be more reactive than others to food additives, pesticides, gluten, corn, and soy. So when you have one of these conditions, it pays to be extra vigilant about your diet to avoid any potential triggers.

Finally, be aware that unrefreshing sleep is a hallmark problem for CFS and fibromyalgia. Please see the Insomnia section on page 212, where I outline strategies to help you learn better sleep habits. After a week or two of practice, we think you'll begin getting the deep, restful slumber that can ease symptoms of both conditions.

Power Up and Lower Pain with Select Supplements

With these conditions, increasing your energy means making sure that your muscles receive the nutrients they need to perform optimally. I advise most people to take a good high-potency multivitamin with minerals. In addition, some studies over the past few years have yielded positive news about the benefits of certain supplements for easing symptoms of fibromyalgia. Though I'm not aware of studies specific to chronic fatigue syndrome and supplements, I believe that the supplements listed below are also likely to be helpful for CFS since many of the same mechanisms are involved for both conditions. Here's what we know.

Vitamin D. We know that low blood levels of vitamin D are common in people with severe pain and also fibromyalgia, but until 2014, researchers hadn't studied whether taking vitamin D supplements might help. In a study published in the journal *Pain*, 30 women with fibromyalgia were given either a placebo or enough vitamin D to raise their blood levels of the vitamin to sufficient levels. After 24 weeks, the women given vitamin D reported that their pain decreased significantly. Since most people have vitamin D deficiencies, especially those living in the northern half of the United States, I recommend taking a daily supplement of 1,000 IU per day.[10]

CoQ10. A deficiency of this proenergy coenzyme has been linked to fibromyalgia. Researchers gave 20 people with fibromyalgia either 300 milligrams of CoQ10 a day or a placebo for 40 days. At the end of the trial, the participants in the CoQ10 group reported less pain, fatigue, and morning tiredness than did the people in the placebo group. What's more, the people who had taken CoQ10 had fewer tender points and less inflammation than did those taking a placebo. I believe people with chronic fatigue syndrome

Start Slow with Chronic Fatigue

Many people with CFS experience something called postexertion malaise, which means that your symptoms might worsen within 12 to 48 hours after you exercise. That's enough to make anyone want to throw in the towel. More exhaustion? No, thank you. But I'm urging you to work through the malaise and keep at it. Here's how.

Start slow. At first, start with just a few minutes of gentle movement and build from there.

Move, then rest. Follow every 1 minute of exercise with 3 minutes of rest. Then increase your exercise sessions slowly by 1 to 5 minutes each session.

Spread it out. Don't feel you have to do all of your exercise at once. It's probably better for you to spread two or three sessions out during the day.

and people with fibromyalgia should take a daily CoQ10 supplement of 200 to 400 milligrams.[11]

Acetyl-l-carnitine (LAC). This so-called nonessential amino acid is found in red meat and dairy products. It plays a role in the production of acetyl-choline, which is a key neurotransmitter; some experts recommend it for memory problems. In a 2007 study, 102 people with fibromyalgia were given either two 500-milligram capsules a day of LAC or a placebo. Researchers tested them at 6 weeks; tender points were reduced in the LAC group, along with other problems, including stiffness, fatigue, and depression.[12, 13]

Move Your Body

When you have fibromyalgia or CFS, the last thing on your mind is exercise. You're exhausted, and you may be in pain. And you also may fear that exercise will worsen your symptoms. What you really want to do is curl up on the couch with your bowlful of treat du jour and binge watch your favorite nighttime soap opera on Netflix.

Please don't. Impossible and counterintuitive as it may seem, one of the best ways to ease either condition is through gentle aerobic exercise. I'm not talking marathons here; I'm talking easy, consistent exercise. Here are a few suggestions:

Try warm water. Warm water exercise is proven to help ease pain in people with fibromyalgia. Your local YMCA may have pool classes for people with arthritis, which are perfect. If not, try other pool-based exercise programs or look into aquatic physical therapy.

Start slowly. Start at a level that's easy for you, and gradually increase the duration and intensity until you're exercising at low to moderate intensity for 20 to 30 minutes two or three times a week.

Don't huff and puff. While you're exercising (and our walking program on page 75 is a perfect way to start), you should be able to speak normally without losing your breath.

Stick with it. Continue regular workouts for at least 1 month before deciding whether or not exercise is improving your symptoms. It's normal that you might feel a little more pain and fatigue at first, but after a couple of weeks, you can expect to feel better.[14]

Cognitive Behavioral Therapy

Cognitive behavioral therapy (CBT) is a talk therapy that helps you change your unhelpful behaviors and thinking. It's been proven as one of the most effective ways for helping people feel better with fibromyalgia, and many experts also believe that this therapy can be a powerful tool for people with chronic fatigue syndrome, too. A 2013 review of 23 studies involving 2,031 people revealed that after 12 weeks, CBT slightly reduced pain, negative mood, and disability, and improvements continued for at least 6 months after therapy ended. To find a therapist near you, visit academyofct.org.[15] Using CBT to manage symptoms by no means suggests that the illness is "all in your head." It teaches you skills that make it easier to cope with the disease.

DR. HOWARD'S Q&A

Q. How do I deal with the depression I get these days? I just don't feel like participating in the same activities I used to enjoy before I developed the pain and fatigue.

A. You can try SAMe (S-adenosylmethionine). Sometimes it takes a fairly large dose, 400 to 800 milligrams daily. Some of the depression that goes with fibromyalgia may be that you have a sluggish thyroid gland, so be sure to have that checked. Make sure you're not eating any foods you might be reacting to. For many people, the reaction includes muscle pain, depression, and anxiety. Start a graded exercise program, and also try EFT—emotional freedom technique. This method can heal past trauma that could be contributing to your illness.

Depression and Anxiety

To *Breakfast at Tiffany's* heroine Holly Golightly, anxiety was "the mean reds." To jazz and soul musicians of all stripes, depression is "the blues." Despite the colorful euphemisms, anxiety and depression are serious and potentially dangerous mental health disorders. And though many effective natural therapies exist to treat these mental health disorders, unfortunately, doctors' treatment of choice—despite the many side effects—are pills.

Though anxiety occurs more often than depression—18 percent of Americans have a diagnosed anxiety disorder, compared to 6 percent who've been diagnosed with depression—depression is the most disabling of all the mental and behavioral disorders.[1, 2]

Do you think you can tell the difference between being chronically anxious and chronically depressed? It's not as black and white as you'd suspect. You might think that anxious people are high-strung and fidgety and that depressed people have low energy and seem sad. But these are stereotypes that cloud the reality and perpetuate the misunderstandings that surround mental illness.

Although anxiety and depression are different medical disorders, they share several similarities. People with depression often feel hopeless and angry. Ordinary daily tasks overwhelm them, and they tend to have low energy levels. People dealing with anxiety can also be overwhelmed by life's responsibilities and may face normal life situations with fear or panic. They, too, can feel chronically exhausted. In fact, many people have aspects of depression *and* anxiety. Both depression and anxiety can interfere with your ability to work or maintain relationships. In severe cases, you may even be unable to leave your house. In conventional medicine, anxiety and depression are usually treated similarly with pills—various antidepressant and antianxiety medications.[3]

Depression: Sadness Squared

Unfortunately, despite all the dramatic drug ads showing depressed people becoming "happy" again once they take the advertised pills, the fact is that

55 to 65 percent of people either don't respond fully to antidepressants or experience side effects, including insomnia, sexual problems, weight gain, restlessness, and memory lapses. More rare but even scarier side effects include suicide, violence, psychosis, and abnormal bleeding.[4]

There's no one-size-fits-all when it comes to depression. You're certainly familiar with the feeling of being sad, unhappy, or even downright miserable. Usually, in someone who doesn't have a diagnosable mental illness, sad feelings are caused by an upsetting event—a death or divorce, a serious illness (yours or a loved one's), a change in financial circumstances, even an "empty nest." The feelings can last a few days, weeks, or a couple of months. But when sadness doesn't go away, and when it interferes with your daily activities, then your depression needs to be addressed. Symptoms of clinical depression include:[5]

- Low mood, most of the time
- Loss of pleasure in daily activities
- Trouble sleeping or sleeping too much
- Changes in appetite—either weight gain or loss
- Exhaustion
- Feelings of worthlessness, self-hate, and guilt
- Difficulty concentrating
- Feeling hopeless
- Suicidal thoughts

Anxiety: When Worry Is Winning

Anxiety comes in a rainbow of variations. At one end of the spectrum is the garden-variety anxiety that we all know so well and experience nearly every day—usually, several times a day. Realities such as the traffic jam, the deadline, the angry boss, the bounced check—all of these can generate anxious feelings. But for most of us, most of the time, these feelings are fleeting; they are your stress-makers. I describe the effects of stress and offer a number of effective stress-relieving remedies in Chapter 5. (You'll find that many of those remedies can also be helpful for depression and anxiety.)

True anxiety, on the other hand, isn't just stress caused by a rotten day. True anxiety is when your stressful feelings become overwhelming, or nearly so, and chronic—you begin to feel as if your life is just one fierce worry after another. That light at the end of the tunnel? You're terrified you'll never see it.

When worry like this consumes you, especially when your worries are unrealistic (your house will burn down during your vacation; the bridge you're driving across will collapse; your airplane could crash; terrorists will bomb your city; you might contract Ebola), then you're edging into the territory of an anxiety disorder. Officially known as generalized anxiety disorder (GAD), this is a very real condition characterized by a very unreal level of worry. When such worry interferes with your daily life, and you've experienced it on a chronic basis for at least 6 months, you need to take action.

Some 6.8 million adults will experience GAD in any given year, according to the Anxiety and Depression Association of America; women are twice as likely as men to be affected.[6] We don't know exactly what causes GAD, but we suspect that genetics, family background, and life experiences, particularly stressful ones, play a role.

Throughout your life, your anxiety levels will shift up or down. If your anxiety levels fall mostly on the mild side of the spectrum, you can enjoy a normal work, family, and social life, though you might find yourself avoiding situations that make you especially anxious (think parties or travel, for example). People with more severe GAD will have trouble dealing with even simple everyday activities.[7]

You may also develop certain physical symptoms, including:[8]

- Muscle tension
- Fatigue
- Restlessness
- Difficulty sleeping
- Irritability
- Edginess

Panic Disorder: Terrifying Feelings Gone Wild

Having a panic attack is a truly terrifying experience. Your heart races; you might have trouble breathing; you break into a sweat. You may even feel chest pain and worry that you're having a heart attack.

Not everyone who experiences a panic attack has a panic disorder—you can have just one attack and never have another. Panic disorder affects some six million people—twice as many women as men; it may be an inherited condition.

Left unaddressed, panic disorder can make you afraid to leave the house (a condition called agoraphobia). Unfortunately, it can be a difficult condition to correctly diagnose. On the good news front, however, once it's diagnosed, panic disorder often responds to treatment, especially to cognitive behavioral therapy and emotional freedom technique (EFT) (see page 106).[9]

When Horror Lingers: Post-Traumatic Stress Disorder (PTSD)

People who have experienced horrific ordeals—combat veterans, victims of violent crimes, survivors of child abuse, or people who have lived through natural disasters, for example—may develop PTSD, which affects nearly eight million Americans. Marked by flashbacks of the event, nightmares, and frightening thoughts, PTSD often causes its sufferers to lose interest in activities they once enjoyed, to become depressed and even feel guilty, and to avoid situations or places that trigger memories of the event. People with PTSD tend to startle easily, have angry outbursts and trouble sleeping, and feel anxious.

A treatment known as accelerated resolution therapy (ART) is a very short-term therapy that researchers at the University of South Florida College of Nursing have studied for its ability to substantially reduce PTSD symptoms, including depression, anxiety, sleep problems, and other issues. They believe that ART could be an effective alternative for traditional PTSD treatments that rely on drugs or lengthy psychotherapy sessions.

This talk therapy uses back-and-forth eye movements as the patient fluctuates between talking about a traumatic scene and using the eye movements to help process the information. As the person integrates memories from traumatic events, he or she replaces painful images by re-envisioning them via a technique called voluntary image replacement. To find a therapist trained in ART, visit acceleratedresolutiontherapy.com.[10, 11]

The Medication Situation

I'll go on record as saying that I'm generally not a big fan of pharmaceuticals as the sole treatment for anxiety and/or depression. All too often, physicians and others in our medical system assume that a chemical imbalance or faulty brain wiring or deficient neurotransmitters are the sole causes of mental disorders. However, that narrow thinking fails to take into account other, easily addressed causes, such as underlying vitamin and mineral deficiencies, allergic reactivity, hormone imbalances, or family dynamics. In my opinion, these all need to be addressed and corrected before the physician prescribes drugs.

However, I do understand that for some people, medication can play a valuable, even lifesaving, role when properly prescribed and carefully monitored. But well before reaching for my prescription pad, I'd make certain that all other factors for a particular patient have been taken into consideration, starting with the basics: diet (including checking for vitamin and mineral deficiencies) and exercise. In my experience, just as food sensitivities can trigger physical problems, they can also play a role in your emotional problems, especially if you're regularly eating foods to which you react.

I have grave concerns about the side effects of psychoactive medicines—many of which might actually worsen the condition you're taking them for, or create other unwanted problems (such as weight gain or loss of sex drive, to name just two). Or they might not work at all, leaving you feeling worse off than when you started. What's more, a recent study showed that a class of drugs frequently prescribed for anxiety, benzodiazepines, could actually play a role in the development of Alzheimer's disease. How's that for an anxiety trigger?[12] Let's take a look at the kinds of drugs that are frequently prescribed for depression and anxiety.

Selective serotonin reuptake inhibitors (SSRIs). These drugs are designed to relieve symptoms by blocking the reabsorption (reuptake) of serotonin by certain nerve cells in the brain. This allows more serotonin to circulate, which may improve your mood. Doctors prescribe these drugs for both anxiety and depression.[13] SSRIs include citalopram (Celexa), escitalopram (Lexapro), fluoxetine (Prozac), paroxetine (Paxil), and sertraline (Zoloft). Among the more common side effects linked to SSRIs are insomnia or its opposite, sleepiness. They're also known to cause weight gain and sexual dysfunction.[14]

Serotonin-norepinephrine reuptake inhibitors (SNRIs). These pills, including venlafaxine (Effexor) and duloxetine (Cymbalta), increase levels of serotonin and another neurotransmitter, norepinephrine. They are considered an appropriate first treatment for anxiety disorders, though they're also prescribed for depression, according to experts at the Anxiety and Depression Association of America.[15, 16]

Both drugs come with a dramatic warning for children, teens, and young adults up to 24 years of age. During clinical studies on antidepressants such as venlafaxine and duloxetine, a small number of people in those age groups became suicidal. We don't know whether that's a side effect of the drug or if depressed young people are simply at higher than normal risk for suicidal thoughts. Still, both drugs are associated with a very long list of side effects, all of which could make a person feel worse rather than better.[17, 18]

Benzodiazepines. These are the drugs formerly known as tranquilizers, back in the *Valley of the Dolls* days. They're prescribed for short-term anxiety treatment because, unlike SNRIs and SSRIs, they act quickly to make you feel relaxed. But these drugs, which include alprazolam (Xanax), clonazepam (Klonopin), diazepam (Valium), and lorazepam (Ativan), also trigger dependence and addiction, and you can develop tolerance to them, meaning that you'll need increasingly higher doses to achieve the same effect.

Benzodiazepines have a huge potential for side effects such as confusion, sleepiness, and even depression. What's more, they're responsible for deadly effects when people drink alcohol while taking them (and opioid painkillers).

According to the Centers for Disease Control and Prevention (CDC), alcohol was involved in about one in five deaths related to abuse of opioid pain relievers or benzodiazepines in 2010. Here's what CDC and FDA researchers found in an analysis of data on drug-related ER visits and deaths.

- Alcohol was involved in 19 percent of the 440,000 ER visits related to opioid abuse and in 27 percent of the 410,000 visits related to benzodiazepine abuse.

- Alcohol was involved in 22 percent of the nearly 4,000 opioid-related deaths and in 21 percent of the 1,500 benzodiazepine-related deaths.[19]

In addition, new research points to another frightening potential outcome of taking benzodiazepines. In a study of nearly 9,000 people over the age of 66, researchers discovered that people who had "ever used" the drugs in the previous 5 years had an increased risk of between 43 to 51 percent for developing Alzheimer's disease.[20] Those findings didn't surprise the research team from the University of Bordeaux in France, however. That's because the same team published a study last year showing that people who used benzodiazepines had a 50 percent higher risk for developing dementia.[21]

My take on this class of drugs is pretty much to avoid them at all costs. Of course, as with everything in medicine, there is the exceptional patient

America's Top-Selling Drug Is an Antipsychotic

I admit it: I was stunned to learn that the drug Abilify (aripiprazole) had become America's top-selling drug in 2013, with sales of *$6,293,801,000.*[22] The drug is prescribed for schizophrenia and bipolar disorder. It is also often prescribed with antidepressants for people diagnosed with depression. Despite the fact that millions of Americans are currently taking Abilify, we don't actually know how it works.[23] In 2012, Richard A. Friedman, MD, professor of psychiatry at Weill Cornell Medical College in New York City, expressed his concern in a *New York Times* article. He wrote that Abilify and similar drugs are increasingly prescribed for people with less serious conditions, such as depression and anxiety—conditions for which they may not be appropriate. I agree. These drugs may have their place in treating serious psychiatric disorders, but I can't imagine the circumstances that would have me prescribe them for less debilitating emotional problems.[24]

in extraordinary circumstances for whom a short-term treatment with these drugs might be appropriate—a physician might rightly prescribe them for someone who has experienced a terribly traumatic event, for example, and then only with appropriate support. The bottom line in my opinion: The use of these drugs should be very carefully considered—and infrequent.

My Natural Approach to Relieving Depression and Anxiety

Though you wouldn't know it from the drug company advertising you see on television and in magazines, the truth is that diet along with many natural therapies can help ease your symptoms of depression or anxiety. Studies show that some of these therapies are every bit as effective as pharmaceutical antidepressants.

The No More Pills Plan Balances Mood Naturally

One key benefit of the No More Pills diet when it comes to depression and anxiety is this: It's extremely low in sugar—in fact, the only sugar it contains comes from fruit and the occasional piece of very dark chocolate, which makes this diet virtually sugar-free. Why is this so important if you're dealing with mood issues?

Because eating sugar can make you feel like you've hopped on a mood roller coaster. Eat that sugary doughnut for breakfast or a midmorning snack and the next thing you know, your mood is going up and down right along with your blood sugar. Soon after downing the doughnut, you're feeling happy as can be. But just a couple hours later, you crash into the doldrums. One key to maintaining a balanced mood is to keep your blood sugar balanced, and that's exactly what the No More Pills diet will do for you. After all, if this type of diet plus exercise, supplements, and stress reduction can reverse Alzheimer's disease, as I described earlier, imagine what it might do to relieve your anxiety and depression. Adding extra servings of the following foods will also help protect your mood.

Fatty fish, such as wild salmon and sardines. As I've mentioned before, fish is rich in omega-3 fatty acids, which studies have shown can ease depression. Aim for at least four servings a week. One 3.5-ounce serving of wild salmon provides about 1,000 to 2,000 milligrams of EPA and DHA, which are the key omega-3s shown to benefit depression. Since most studies show you need to take about 2 grams of fish oil a day, I also recommend that you take a good fish oil supplement.[25]

Enjoy foods rich in B vitamins. I've seen several studies that point to the mood-lifting benefits of the B-vitamin group, so concentrate on eating plenty of foods that contain B_6, $B_{12,}$ and folate. You'll find these in leafy green veggies; organic eggs; and organic fish, chicken, and meat.[26]

Talk Therapy for Depression and Anxiety

For many of my patients who have anxiety or depression (or both), once I work on identifying any food allergies and help them structure a more appropriate diet, I usually suggest they also engage in some form of talk therapy. One of the best studied and most effective of these is cognitive behavioral therapy.

Cognitive behavioral therapy (CBT) has been proven effective in hundreds of clinical trials for many different mental disorders. It's different from the psychotherapy you probably think of first—the Woody Allen lying-on-the-couch-Freudian-style, where you pour out your past experiences to a therapist over months or years, seeking the aha moments that help you understand why you behave the way you do. Instead, a CBT therapist will teach you how to create new and more useful thought and behavior patterns. The therapist will also help you to identify your distressing thoughts and to figure out whether or not those thoughts are distorted—and will show you how distorted thinking can affect your behavior.

Once the therapist helps you see that your thoughts are distorted, the therapist will help you learn to change the distorted thinking. When people think more realistically, say CBT experts, they feel better. The therapy then focuses on teaching you how to solve problems and create more helpful behaviors.[27]

The process is goal-oriented: Most CBT therapists will help you develop a goal list and decide which goals you'll work on yourself and which you'll work out in therapy. The therapist will also help you develop an action plan or homework to do during the week. To find a CBT therapist near you, visit academyofct.org.[28]

In a CBT study published in the September 2014 issue of *Lancet Psychiatry*, researchers analyzed 101 clinical trials, which included more than 13,000 participants. They compared the effectiveness of various pharmaceutical drugs and different psychotherapies for treating social anxiety disorder (the fear or anxiety of being in social situations).[29, 30]

The research team concluded that one-on-one cognitive behavioral therapy might prove more effective than drugs for treating adults who have social anxiety disorder. What's more, they said, it has fewer side effects and "should be regarded as the best intervention for initial treatment" of the disorder.[31]

Mood Improvement via Movement

You've certainly heard of the "runner's high." It's what happens in your brain when you exercise. You release feel-good, natural, pain-killing chemicals called endorphins. Researchers have discovered that exercise, particularly

Is What We Think about Serotonin All Wrong?

Serotonin is a brain chemical that many antidepressant/antianxiety drugs have been developed to target because of the role we think it plays in depression. Though the pharmaceutical industry has focused its depression treatment attention on creating drugs that increase levels of serotonin, the fact is, we still don't know whether decreased levels of serotonin actually contribute to depression; it could be that depression itself decreases serotonin levels.[32]

Serotonin's job (another neurotransmitter, norepinephrine, also plays a key role) is to transmit nerve signals from one brain cell to another. Since the late 1980s, brain scientists have theorized that increasing serotonin levels is key to treating depression. The well-known drug Prozac (fluoxetine), a selective serotonin reuptake inhibitor (SSRI) intended to increase serotonin levels, came to market in the 1980s, and after its introduction came scores of newer drugs with various negative side effects. These drugs created a king's ransom of profits for the pharmaceutical industry.

What's fascinating about the way Prozac catapulted into popularity isn't that it was so much more effective than the antidepressants it replaced. Instead, its popularity with prescribers was because it caused fewer side the kind that gets your heart pumping, can decrease tension, elevate and stabilize mood, improve your sleep—and even give your self-esteem a boost.[33]

Fortunately, you don't have to become a gym rat to achieve these uplifting benefits—even a 10-minute walk around the block can work the same mood-boosting magic as a 45-minute workout. And, say researchers, exercise works fast to ease depression. Just a brisk walk can deliver several hours of relief, say experts at the Anxiety and Depression Association of America. On the other hand, pharmaceuticals often take 4 to 6 weeks to become effective.[34]

What's more, physically active people have lower rates of anxiety and depression than sedentary people do. In one study, researchers discovered that people who exercised regularly were 25 percent less likely to develop depression or an anxiety disorder over the next 5 years.[35]

effects than did the previous generation of drugs, such as tricyclics, which also targeted serotonin levels, among other actions.[36]

Today, studies show that taking Prozac or similar drugs doesn't help 60 to 70 percent of people who have depression.[37] And now, a new study hints that everything we think we know about serotonin and its role in depression could be wrong. A team of researchers at the VA Medical Center and the Wayne State University School of Medicine in Detroit set out to investigate the role, if any, serotonin plays in depression. To do so, they bred a strain of mice that was unable to produce serotonin. Then the researchers tested these mice for symptoms of depression (yes, even mice can be depressed). Though the mice behaved more compulsively and aggressively, they weren't depressed.

The researchers stressed the mice with various tests and saw that normal mice and serotonin-free mice behaved the same way under stress. The researchers also learned that antidepressant medications lessened depression—to the same extent—in both normal and serotonin-free mice. So their theory is that serotonin may not, in fact, have such a dominant role in depression after all. The researchers expect that their discovery will trigger a new wave of research in the development of antidepressants.[38]

My advice to you is this: Find some activity you love; it doesn't have to be "exercise," per se—it can be gardening, housework (though most people I know don't find that much fun), or running around after your active children or grandchildren. Just moving for 30 minutes or so most days of the week will go a long way toward relieving depression and anxiety.

Traditional Chinese Medicine

As a physician who practices integrative medicine, I have been trained in and employ a variety of evidence-based therapies, choosing those that best suit each individual I treat. But I'd have to say my go-to choice for treating anxiety and depression is often traditional Chinese medicine (TCM). Throughout this book, I discuss the effectiveness of acupuncture for a number of different conditions, and you're probably aware that acupuncture is one of the therapies under the TCM umbrella. But TCM is much more than just acupuncture—it encompasses medicinal herbs, massage, diet, movement, meditation, and breathing exercises.

In TCM, healers use herbs much differently than most Western herbalists do. Rarely are Chinese herbs used singly, nor are they typically used to treat single symptoms. That's because TCM practitioners believe that symptoms are caused by a variety of imbalances within your system that block the flow of *qi*, or your vital energy, so often herbs are blended specifically to correct those imbalances. Sometimes practitioners will blend herbs for each patient; sometimes they will use classic Chinese herb blends.

For treating depression and anxiety, I often rely on a few Chinese herbal formulas that belong to a category known as herbs that "nourish the heart and calm the spirit." I just love the names of these blends. They're an indication of how differently TCM views medicine. You certainly won't find bottles of Heavenly Emperor, Peaceful Spirit, or Restful Sleep at your corner drugstore! If you want to explore TCM and Chinese herbs, I recommend that you find a certified TCM practitioner (this is not a DIY therapy). Visit the National Certification Commission for Acupuncture and Oriental Medicine at nccaom.org.[39]

Supplements That Ease Anxiety and Depression

Before I would recommend pharmaceutical pills for treating depression and anxiety, I would suggest you take these supplements. None of these works overnight, so give them at least a couple of months to see if they affect your mood for the better.

Theanine for anxiety relief. L-theanine is an amino acid that's been studied for several different effects; most of the research centers on its effectiveness as an anxiety treatment. It's something I use first for many patients, especially because it doesn't interact with other medications they may be taking. Theanine is found mainly in green and black teas, and you can find it in supplement form at health food stores and some drugstores. In studies, it seems to relax the mind without causing drowsiness.[40] In one study, taking 400 milligrams a day of theanine reduced anxiety among people with schizophrenia. A cup of black tea has about 20 milligrams of theanine.[41]

Boost mood with B vitamins. We know that vitamin deficiencies can cause mental problems. For example, thiamin, or vitamin B_1, deficiency is directly connected with depression. Like other B-complex vitamins, thiamin is sometimes called an antistress vitamin because it may strengthen the immune system and improve the body's ability to withstand stressful conditions.[42] And Finnish researchers found that high to normal blood levels of vitamin B_{12} increased the effectiveness of drugs and therapy in 115 people with depression. Other studies suggest that getting enough vitamin B_{12} may prevent depression in the first place.[43] My advice? Take a B-complex vitamin once a day.

Fish oil may ease depression. The latest research shows that taking fish oil can increase certain white blood cells that gobble up inflammatory substances. And that might play a role in the fact that fish oil seems to be useful for easing depression, which some researchers suspect has an inflammatory component.[44] I like NOW Foods Ultra Omega-3. It doesn't have a fishy aftertaste; it's mercury-free; and it contains $2\frac{1}{2}$ times the usual EPA/DHA dose in each capsule. Most fish oil capsules have 300 milligrams of combined EPA/DHA in a single 1,000-milligram (1-gram) capsule. Ultra Omega-3 has 750 milligrams of combined EPA/DHA in one 1,000-milligram capsule. I recommend one to three capsules a day.

SAMe: Depression relief equal to pharmaceuticals. SAMe, which is short for S-adenosylmethionine, is a naturally occurring compound made from an amino acid. Your body uses it to produce neurotransmitters, and it's possible that it may boost levels of serotonin and dopamine. In Europe, SAMe has been prescribed as a treatment for depression for more than

25 years. A recent report from the Agency for Healthcare Research and Quality analyzed the results of 28 studies and found that SAMe was about as effective as standard antidepressants, sans the side effects. The one downside of SAMe, however, is its price. It could cost up to $200 per month, depending on the dose you need. On the bright side, it may also relieve arthritis and other forms of pain. Doses range from 400 to 1,600 milligrams per day,[45] but most people do well on the 400-milligram daily dose.

New research on curcumin for depression/anxiety. The potent antioxidant compound curcumin, which is found in the Indian spice turmeric, was recently proven in a clinical trial to be helpful for relieving depression. In this gold standard 2014 study, published in the *Journal of Affective Disorders,* 56 people diagnosed with major depressive disorder were treated with a curcumin extract (500 milligrams twice a day) or a placebo. Participants were asked to rate their depression levels on a standardized scale. By Week 4, continuing through Week 8, curcumin was significantly more effective than the placebo in lowering symptoms. What's more, noted the researchers, curcumin was even more effective in relieving symptoms of atypical depression, which they said is a more difficult disorder to treat.[46]

"Curcumin promotes the formation of new brain cells, a process called neurogenesis," says Ajay Goel, PhD, director of epigenetics and cancer prevention at Baylor Research Institute in Dallas. What's more, he says, curcumin inhibits monoamine oxidase, which helps boost the levels of various neurotransmitters to help fight depression. It might also play a role in easing anxiety, theorizes Dr. Goel. "I believe taking curcumin could help treat anxiety, because anxiety is also a consequence of altered levels of various neurotransmitters." The extract used in the study is known as BCM-95, which is available in several supplements, including Life Extension Super Bio-Curcumin and Curamin.[47]

German chamomile: Gentle relief from anxiety. Chamomile (*Matricaria recutita*) is an excellent herb for people whose anxiety upsets their digestion. It contains compounds that relieve spasms in the gut as well as volatile oils that have sedative qualities. In one 2012 University of Pennsylvania study, researchers gave 57 people diagnosed with anxiety, depression, or both either a chamomile extract or a placebo for 8 weeks. The researchers concluded that chamomile effectively reduced their symptoms. The dose was four 220-milligram capsules a day. A similar extract to the one used in the study is Nature's Way standardized chamomile.[48, 49]

● ●

DR. HOWARD'S Q&A

Q. I often feel terribly sad as soon as daylight savings time ends. My MD wants me to take an antidepressant. Is there an alternative? I hate taking pills.

A. Sad? Get a SAD light. (SAD stands for seasonal affective disorder—it's a real problem for many people.) A number of studies prove that light therapy can ease depression triggered by the dark days of winter. One of my favorite reasonably priced lights is the SunTouch Plus by Nature Bright.

Diabetes

When you hear the words *terrifying epidemic,* the first thing you envision is a disease like Ebola, which was capturing daily headlines and nightly television news stories around the country as I was writing this book. In December 2014, the Centers for Disease Control and Prevention reported that worldwide, nearly 6,400 people, mostly from West African countries, had died.[1, 2, 3]

Compare that to diabetes. In 2010, diabetes was the seventh leading cause of death in the United States. It was listed as the cause of death on more than 69,000 death certificates and as a contributing cause on 234,000 additional death certificates that same year. In 2012, almost 30 million Americans had diabetes—that's 9.3 percent of the population, nearly one in every 10 people. Of Americans 65 and older, almost 26 percent have diabetes. Diabetes contributes to blindness, amputations, heart disease, kidney disease, neuropathy, Alzheimer's disease, and dementia, among other painful and life-shortening conditions. That's what I call a truly terrifying epidemic.[4]

And the worst thing about those numbers? Type 2 diabetes, the far more prevalent form of the disease, is largely preventable.

Why this astounding epidemic? I reviewed many of the reasons back in Chapter 1. In a nutshell, it's our couch potato lifestyle married to our factory farm/big food/big pharma culture. We are growing the nutrition right out of our produce and our livestock. We are polluting our waters and our atmosphere. We are concocting processed foods out of unhealthy and downright harmful chemicals. Our jobs are largely sedentary, and we're addicted to sitting and staring into the screens of our TVs, computers, tablets, and cell phones.

And to the "rescue" comes the pharmaceutical industry with its expensive drugs, riddled with side effects, to treat illnesses that, like diabetes, should be—and could be—prevented.

Don't mistake my message. I'm not saying that all drugs are harmful or that they aren't important tools for treating many conditions. Under the right circumstances, certain drugs are essential. I am saying, however, that taking pills as the first and only line of defense for treating lifestyle diseases, like diabetes, makes no sense to me whatsoever, especially when some of those pills actually worsen the disease, contribute to causing other diseases, and certainly never offer the hope of a cure. In fact, once diagnosed, you're usually condemned to a lifetime of pill taking.

The Downside of Diabetes Drugs

I'm not alone in worrying about the problems that come from medicating people with diabetes, especially when they're in the early stages of the disease. A 2014 study published in the journal *JAMA Internal Medicine* found that for many people the benefits of taking diabetes medications are so small that they're outweighed by the minor harms and risks associated with treatment. The authors of that study strongly urge us to change the root causes of the diabetes epidemic rather than to medicate otherwise healthy patients with so-called prediabetes.[5]

"Ultimately, the aim of a treatment is not to lower blood sugar for its own sake, but to prevent debilitating or deadly complications" of the disease, says John S. Yudkin, MD, the study coauthor and emeritus professor of medicine at University College London.

How old people are when they begin taking diabetes pills, plus the hassles and side effects of the treatment, are important factors as to whether or not they'll benefit from taking a drug. That's the conclusion Dr. Yudkin and his team came to as a result of their 20-year study of type 2 diabetes treatments, involving more than 5,000 people in the United Kingdom. Lowering blood sugar played a far less important role as a benefit, he says.[6]

And there's this: The top-selling drug, metformin, is considered the frontline treatment for type 2 diabetes. In fact, in a 2012 study published in *Diabetes Care*, researchers suggested that doctors should also expand the pool of people who should take metformin to those diagnosed with prediabetes.

Here's the worrisome downside: In a 2013 study also published in *Diabetes Care*, researchers linked metformin use to impaired cognitive function.[7, 8]

Diabetes 101

Type 2 diabetes occurs when your cells become resistant to the hormone insulin. Insulin, produced in a cone-shaped organ called the pancreas, is the key that "unlocks" your cells to let in glucose, or blood sugar, which cells depend on for energy. When cells start resisting insulin's action and don't "unlock," the pancreas pumps out increasingly higher levels of insulin. When you can't produce enough insulin to meet increased demands, blood sugar rises and type 2 diabetes develops.

It may sound like a benign condition to you—so what, my blood has too much sugar in it? How can that hurt me? Here's how: High sugar levels in the blood weaken your blood vessels—and your heart. As an easy metaphor, think of that sugar as a tiny sharp-edged diamond, ping-ponging through your vessels, damaging vessel walls. High blood sugar weakens blood vessels and, especially when combined with high blood pressure and high blood fats, leads to heart attacks, strokes, and peripheral artery disease. It gradually shuts down the vulnerable vessels of the kidneys and the eyes, causing kidney failure and blindness. Left untreated, diabetes compromises your entire circulatory system, which in turn slows wound healing, makes infections more difficult to overcome, and eventually creates the kind of circulation problems that can lead to nerve damage, diabetic ulcers, and even amputations.[9]

Type 1 diabetes, which accounts for about 5 percent of all diabetes cases, is an autoimmune disease. With this type of diabetes, your immune system attacks and destroys the beta cells in the pancreas, which produce insulin. People with type 1 diabetes must monitor blood sugar carefully and give themselves insulin injections, or use an insulin pump.[10]

Who's at Risk?

Several factors are commonly recognized by doctors as putting you at risk for type 2 diabetes. They include:

- Family history
- Being over age 45
- Being overweight or obese
- Having blood pressure higher than 140/90 mm Hg

- Having HDL (good) cholesterol levels lower than 35 mg/dL or a triglyceride level above 250 mg/dL
- Having impaired fasting glucose, impaired glucose tolerance, or fasting blood sugar levels above 100 mg/dL
- Waist measurement more than 35 inches for women and 40 inches for men
- Sedentary lifestyle

Look at this list carefully. What is missing? FOOD! Are you kidding me? I think it's shocking that the number one, most obvious diabetes risk factor is missing from that list, and it's the diet that most Americans are eating these days, called the standard American diet (SAD). In fact, more than a decade ago, leading researchers from Harvard University published their study proving that our "Western-style diet" has increased the incidence of diabetes.[11] And a 2013 study published in the *American Journal of Medicine* confirms the connection: Following a Western-style diet leads to greater risk of diabetes, heart disease, and premature death, says study author Tasnime Akbaraly, PhD, a research fellow at University College London.[12]

How to Stop Diabetes Before It Starts

You're in your doctor's office, and she's going over the results of your recent checkup, which included routine blood tests. She has some news that you're not too happy to hear. Namely, that you've gained some weight since your last checkup and your blood sugar, cholesterol, and blood pressure have edged above normal limits. According to your doctor, you have prediabetes.

A prediabetes diagnosis occurs when your blood sugar levels measure 100 to 125 mg/dL or your A1C (a measurement of blood sugar over time) is 5.7 to 6.4. If your blood sugar levels are 126 mg/dL or above or your A1C is 6.5 or above, the diagnosis is type 2 diabetes.

If you're wondering why your doctor is diagnosing you with a condition before you even *have* that condition, you're not alone. You might think it means that you're at extremely high risk for developing diabetes—to the extent that maybe it makes good sense to take a pill now in hopes of staving off the disease.

The truth is, less than 50 percent of all people who are diagnosed with prediabetes actually develop diabetes within 10 years. And yet, quite often as the first line of defense, your doctor might suggest a pill, usually the antidiabetes drug metformin.

Here's the wrong reaction to getting a prediabetes diagnosis: "Whew, at least I don't have diabetes," says Matt Longjohn, MD, MPH, who is the national health officer for the YMCA of the USA.[13] "Your reaction really should be, 'Wow—I need to do something about this *right now,*'" he says.

One smart and scientifically proven way to stop prediabetes in its tracks, and prevent it from becoming the real deal, is to join the coach-led weight loss program called the Diabetes Prevention Program. Conducted at YMCAs around the country, the program can prevent nearly 60 percent of people with prediabetes from developing diabetes. If you're over age 60, that number rises to 71 percent, says Dr. Longjohn.

People in the YMCA program typically meet for 16 weekly hour-long classes led by a specially trained lifestyle coach. The coach helps instill healthy, diabetes-protective behaviors by teaching how to eat more healthfully and that exercise is vital to preventing diabetes. In the program, people either participate or take metformin. Twice as many people who took the course prevented diabetes, compared to the metformin group.[14] To find a program near you, check the YMCA Web site,[15] or visit the CDC.gov Web site and type "diabetes prevention program" into the search box.[16]

How the No More Pills Plan
Defeats Diabetes

If you have risk factors for diabetes or have been diagnosed with it, you have the right book in your hands. The No More Pills Plan is the ideal diet for preventing diabetes or helping reduce its severity. Why? *Because the plan is extremely low in carbohydrates.* Low-carb diets like this plan should be the first line of attack for treatment of type 2 diabetes and should also be used (in conjunction with insulin) for people who have type 1 diabetes, according to the findings of a July 2014 study published in the journal *Nutrition.*[17]

A team of 26 physicians and nutrition researchers pored through mountains of previously published research and came up with key points that highlight why low-carb diets can reliably reduce high blood sugar, slash diabetes risk, and also reduce the risk for heart disease. Here are just some of the points released by the research team based on their study.

- People with type 2 diabetes on low-carb diets can reduce and frequently even eliminate their medications. People with type 1 diabetes on low-carb diets usually require less insulin.
- Compared to the side effects of pharmaceuticals for diabetes, lowering blood sugar levels via a low-carb diet has no side effects.
- High blood sugar is the most important feature of diabetes. Restricting carbohydrates has the greatest effect on reducing blood glucose levels.
- Our obesity and type 2 diabetes epidemics have occurred because calorie increases in our diets are almost entirely due to eating more carbohydrates.
- You don't even have to lose weight—restricting your carbohydrate intake is enough to achieve health benefits.
- Although weight loss is not required for the diabetes benefits, carbohydrate restriction is the best diet for weight loss.
- A low-carb diet for people with type 2 diabetes is at least as good as other diet interventions, and frequently it is much better.
- Replacing carbs with proteins is generally beneficial to people with diabetes.
- Dietary total and saturated fats do not raise the risk of heart disease.
- Carbohydrates have more to do with raising triglyceride levels than dietary fats do.
- A low-carbohydrate diet is the most effective method of reducing triglyceride levels and raising levels of healthy HDL cholesterol.

Lower Blood Sugar with Food and Drink Secrets

Once people who have high blood sugar start on the No More Pills Plan, they typically find that their blood sugar drops after a month or two. I also like adding these smart tricks, all of which have been scientifically proven to help lower blood sugar.

No More Needles for Mary Zuk

Last February, Mary Zuk, 73, came to see me in Chicago (she was a long way from her hometown in Ocean Isle Beach, North Carolina). She had a long list of worrisome issues: Her diabetes was out of control, she had abdominal pain, and she had bouts of diarrhea after eating. A previous doctor told her she was lactose intolerant, but the recommended Lactaid milk didn't help.

She was an insulin-dependent diabetic. But despite the insulin and an oral antidiabetes pill, her blood sugar was all over the place, swinging from 94 one morning to 290 the next. We tested her for allergies and learned she was reactive to aspartame, MSG, sulfites, grain alcohols, cane sugar, corn, and dairy.

I advised her to avoid all her allergenic foods and recommended a No More Pills–style diet and exercise. I gave her the corn-free multivitamin Perque 2, NOW Foods Ultra Omega-3 fish oil, and a Renew Life probiotic with 50 billion organisms in each capsule. We set up a phone consult for March, after she was back home.

When we spoke in March, just 1 month after our first visit, Mary was happy. By removing additives, dyes, artificial sugars, cane sugar, corn, dairy, and gluten from her diet, she found that her fasting glucose had gone from 299 to 69 in a month. Her doctor in North Carolina was amazed. She was still taking one oral antidiabetic pill, but no longer needed the insulin. Plus, she'd lost 8 pounds.

Mary called again in April. "It's been fabulous. You have changed my life," she told me. Her A1C (a measure of long-term glucose levels) was down from 8.5 to 7.0. She was still taking just one antidiabetic pill and no insulin.

I called Mary again in October to follow up. She said, "I feel really good if I follow my diet." Her A1C had stayed down at 7.2 despite a bout of pneumonia. She said she had lost a total of 60 pounds, was still off insulin, and was taking her one antidiabetes pill. She said, "It's like a miracle. People keep telling me how wonderful I look."

Have a shot of vinegar with starchy meals. Though you won't be eating many high-glycemic foods while you're on this plan, there's always the chance that you'll want to splurge when Aunt Nicolina invites you over for her lasagna Bolognese on your birthday. When you indulge, keep your blood sugar from spiking by having a tablespoon of vinegar in a green salad along with the starchy entrée, or even in a quick vinegar shooter (mixed with seltzer, it makes a refreshing spritzer). This trick can lower your postmeal blood sugar by 42 percent, says Stavros Liatis, MD, consultant in internal medicine and diabetes at Laiko Hospital in Athens, Greece. According to Dr. Liatis, who studied the effects of vinegar on blood sugar, "The addition of vinegar might be one of many weapons to fight high blood sugar."

Drink your coffee. It turns out that people who drink the most coffee have the lowest diabetes risk. If you drink three or more cups a day, you have a 37 percent lower risk than people who drink just one.[18]

Nibble some nuts. A 2014 study published in the journal *Nutrition* compared people who ate a couple of servings of pistachio nuts a day to those who did not eat nuts. People in the pistachio group lowered their markers for metabolic syndrome and reduced inflammation levels.[19] (I love to use pistachios as "croutons" in my salad.) In other tasty news, almonds and walnuts have also been studied and proven to help lower blood sugar.[20]

Savor some strawberries. They're sweet, yummy, and low in sugar, and they pack a little blood sugar–lowering power, too, according to two 2012 studies. Because strawberries are a powerhouse antioxidant fruit, they also lower markers of inflammation. Choose deeply colored, organic-only strawberries and enjoy. Ounce for ounce, they contain more vitamin C than oranges.[21]

These Supplements Lower Blood Sugar

Lots of supplements promise that they can help lower your blood sugar. In my experience, these are the ones that really work.

Add some magnesium. This mineral is a key player in bodily functions ranging from protein synthesis to blood pressure regulation. What's more, it can improve sensitivity to insulin and can lower blood sugar in people with type 2 diabetes.

Dose: 200 to 250 milligrams twice a day; avoid magnesium if you have advanced kidney disease.[22]

Reach for ALA. Alpha-lipoic acid is an antioxidant that performs triple duty for people with diabetes: It improves numbness and nerve pain, which eases diabetic neuropathy, and it can lower blood sugar and help with insulin control.

Dose: Start with 300 milligrams twice a day.

Chill inflammation with fish oil. The latest research shows that taking fish oil can increase certain white blood cells that gobble up inflammatory substances. While chronic inflammation is linked to insulin resistance, the main driver behind type 2 diabetes, fish oil has not been shown to actually improve insulin resistance.[23] I recommend NOW Foods Ultra Omega-3, which has 750 milligrams of combined EPA/DHA in one 1,000-milligram capsule. Take one to three capsules a day.

Win with the red wine supplement. Resveratrol, a compound found in red wine, improves blood sugar levels in people with type 2 diabetes, according to two recent studies. In one 2014 study, participants who took 200 milligrams of resveratrol for 26 weeks lowered their A1C scores compared with those who took a placebo. They also had better memory performance, which is certainly a nice bonus. In a 2012 study, after 3 months of taking a 250-milligram resveratrol supplement, participants with type 2 diabetes had lower A1C scores, lower blood pressure (a drop of about 12 points, systolic), and lower cholesterol.[24, 25]

Exercise Is Everything

When it comes to beating diabetes, you'll need to combine the No More Pills diet with exercise to maximize your chances for lowering the dosage of your medications or, better still, getting off the pills. In fact, exercise has been proven to be as effective as medication for beating type 2 diabetes. That's because when you exercise, glucose leaves the bloodstream and enters muscle cells as fuel. The more muscle you build, the more glucose your muscles can store—thus dropping the glucose levels in your blood. As an added benefit, once you add exercise to your daily schedule, you'll likely lose a few pounds, which will improve your insulin response, and that will also help lower blood sugar.

Here are two smart exercise strategies that are specifically designed to improve diabetes.

1. **Focus on interval training.** I mentioned this in Chapter 4, but it's especially helpful for people with diabetes. One study showed that when you alternate high-intensity bursts of aerobic activity for a couple of minutes with low-intensity rest periods for as little as 10 minutes of total activity (via an exercise bike, an elliptical machine, or good old-fashioned walking), you can lower glucose levels by 13 percent for up to 24 hours. Aim for 90 minutes a week.

2. **Add some weight.** People who do a combination of strength training and aerobics can lower their A1C by 1 percent—which translates to a 20 percent lower risk for developing heart disease and a 40 percent lower chance of eye or kidney disease. No pill can do that!

   No access to a gym or equipment? No problem! Just doing simple bodyweight exercises, such as pushups, lunges, and squats, can help. Aim to do one or two sets of each move at least twice a week for 20 minutes.[26]

• •

DR. HOWARD'S Q&A

Q. When I test my own blood sugar after I come back from the gym, it's always higher than it should be. That makes no sense to me. What could be the reason for this?

A. You may be stressed by your exercise! Feeling stressed can raise your cortisol levels and therefore your blood sugar. I see people running into health clubs looking harried, pushing themselves through a routine, and then rushing to get showered, dressed, and on to the next (overscheduled) activity. Be sure to make your exercise something you actually enjoy doing, and schedule adequate time to do it!

Eczema and Psoriasis

Redness, itching, scaling, peeling, cracking—these are the painful signs of troubled skin. Two common skin problems responsible for symptoms like these are eczema and psoriasis. Both bedevil—and, in the worst cases, even disfigure—millions and millions of people.

Eczema is an umbrella diagnosis for a variety of rashes that are caused by allergies to something in your environment or your diet. Psoriasis causes skin to thicken and scale when skin cell growth goes haywire and forms inflamed patches, often on the elbows, knees, scalp, and other areas. Up to 30 percent of people with psoriasis also experience joint pain.

Standard medical treatment for both conditions is similar and often starts with prescription steroid creams. Using the steroid skin products can calm the skin reaction for a while, but when you stop using the cream, the cause of the skin problem is still there and the rash returns. In addition, prolonged use of steroids has a harmful side effect: They can thin the skin.

As far as I'm concerned, both eczema and psoriasis are usually delayed-type allergy "inside job" problems, misdiagnosed and mistreated as skin diseases. Rubbing ointments and creams on the skin or taking immunosuppressant drugs won't do the job, because these methods don't treat the root problem. To do that, you have to identify which food proteins—often casein (dairy)—are responsible for the problem, and then you have to remove them from your diet.[1, 2]

What's more, using steroids on your skin while you continue to eat foods to which you're allergic is just like feeding the fire on one side while you try to put it out on the other. Using immunosuppressant drugs, such as cyclosporine or methotrexate, which are often prescribed for psoriasis and eczema, is even more inappropriate and dangerous (not to mention expensive—these can cost up to $10,000 a year). To me, this perfectly illustrates bad medicine, in which you quell the inflammatory fire with dangerous and expensive pills—instead of treating the root problem. I've even known doctors to recommend Aveeno products (main ingredient, oats) to people to help soothe their eczema or psoriasis. But many people are actually allergic to oats! If you're one of them, the last thing you want to do is to apply oats to already irritated skin.

Let There Be Light—Therapy

Several types of light therapy are prescribed for skin problems. One that I've seen work is UVB therapy (narrow-band ultraviolet light B). I have a 65-year-old female patient who had psoriasis lesions on her arms, legs, and trunk for many years. She'd used steroid creams, but they weren't very effective. Finally, I suggested she stop eating dairy, gluten, and corn and begin UVB therapy. At my suggestion, she also took some Ayurvedic detox treatments with herbs and sesame oil. Happily, this combination approach was highly effective for her—now, her skin is almost completely clear. She continues with occasional UV light treatments and follows the No More Pills Plan. You can get a prescription for UVB light devices for home use from a dermatologist.[3]

The No More Pills Plan for Healthy Skin

Healing eczema and psoriasis comes down to identifying and eliminating the food triggers to which you're allergic—via the No More Pills Plan—as well as eliminating any environmental allergens that could be contributing to your skin problems.

I have successfully treated literally hundreds of people with eczema and psoriasis by identifying and eliminating allergens from their diets and surroundings. So the first thing I recommend to people who have skin problems is to go on an elimination diet or have the tests done to pinpoint which foods or substances might be causing their reactions.

Another major benefit of the No More Pills Plan is that it successfully reduces inflammation, which plays such a huge role in skin problems. On this plan, you are eating the healthy fats you need to quell skin problems, and you are getting plenty of free-radical-fighting antioxidants, too.

Research confirms the benefits of following an anti-inflammatory diet when you have skin problems, says Rajani Katta, MD, professor of dermatology at Baylor College of Medicine in Houston. In her research paper, "Diet and Dermatology: The Role of Dietary Intervention in Skin Disease," published in 2014, she mentions a study in which a Mediterranean diet, which shares many aspects of the No More Pills Plan, lowered participants' inflammation markers. Dr. Katta also said that people with psoriasis should increase their intake of fruits and vegetables, limit sugar and saturated fat, and emphasize eating foods "in their natural state over highly processed foods." And that's exactly what I have in mind for you.

Foods That Help Heal Skin Problems

Eat three to five daily servings of these carotenoid-rich fruits and vegetables.

- Carrots
- Deep green, leafy vegetables
- Mangoes
- Sweet potatoes
- Tomatoes
- Winter squash

Eat at least five weekly servings of omega-3-rich fish, including:

- Arctic char
- Black cod (sablefish)
- Herring
- Mussels
- Oysters
- Wild salmon
- Sardines

Smart Supplement Strategies to Improve Your Skin

When I start working with someone who has eczema or psoriasis, I recommend that they take these four key supplements. The anti-inflammatory power these exert can help speed your way to clearer skin.

Probiotics. One of the first supplements I recommend for anyone with eczema or psoriasis is probiotics. That's because most people with these conditions have gut irritation from years of eating foods to which they have delayed-type food allergies. Taking probiotics can help restore function and health to the gut and can help blunt inflammation. I like Renew Life Ultimate Flora Senior Formula, which contains 30 billion colony-forming units. Take one capsule twice daily with a light meal.

Berberine. This plant alkaloid is found in Oregon grape, goldenseal, and barberry, among other plants. It has a long history of use in Ayurvedic and traditional Chinese medicine and is believed to have anti-inflammatory action. Studies show that ointments containing berberine help improve eczema and psoriasis. Take 500 milligrams of berberine capsules one to two times a day. I like the Thorne brand.[4, 5, 6]

Fish oil. Several studies have shown that high doses of fish oil improve psoriasis, and at least one recent study shows that high-dose fish oil therapy significantly improves eczema symptoms, as well. Try NOW Foods Ultra Omega-3 fish oil softgel capsules, which contain 500 milligrams of EPA

How to Find Safer Skin Care Products

Most drugstore or beauty shop body products are loaded with allergens and chemicals. Just read the labels on soaps, lotions, shampoos, and conditioners, and you'll see what I mean: potentially toxic chemicals like sodium laureth (sodium laureth sulfate), methylparaben, propylparaben, and polyethylene glycol (PEG).

The Environmental Working Group, a nonprofit organization, has a Web site at ewg.org that lets you find out if your beauty products contain potentially allergenic or otherwise harmful chemicals. They even offer a handy smartphone app you can download and take shopping.[7]

But it's not just toxic chemicals that are problematic. For some people, even so-called natural ingredients can trigger skin reactions. Some beauty and skin care products contain common food allergens, such as hydrolyzed wheat protein, oat protein, milk protein, and corn syrup. If you have eczema or psoriasis, you need to avoid these.

How to do it? Moisturize with simple oils, such as organic olive or coconut oil, or with allergen-free body products. My favorites are from Acure and Andalou. Dr. Bronner's makes a great old-fashioned soap in either liquid or bar form. My favorite is their fragrance-free bar, but they also have several natural scents—peppermint, almond, rose, citrus, lavender, and tea tree oil. (Even though these are made from organic ingredients, you could still be allergic, so discontinue the use of any of these if they worsen your skin.)

and 250 milligrams of DHA in each gelcap. Take seven gelcaps a day—two with breakfast, two with lunch, and three with dinner.

Vitamin D. Since light (sunshine, too) helps improve skin conditions such as psoriasis and eczema, then it stands to reason that the "sunshine vitamin" might also help improve them. That's been confirmed, though, in a

Elaine's Clear-Skin Plan

Elaine Rosenblatt, 63, of Chicago, was at her wit's end—nothing she tried would calm the red patches that inflamed her skin. The worst inflammation was right on her face, plus her eyes were crusted with yellow fluid. Medication, including antihistamines, had done no good. Along with her skin problems, she had sinus congestion, and nasal sprays weren't helping, either. She had tested positive for antinuclear antibodies (ANA), and her doctor suspected she could have an autoimmune disorder, so he referred her to a rheumatologist. Instead, she came to see me.

I tested her and discovered that she had delayed-type allergies to many different foods—gluten, dairy, white potatoes, white vinegar, oats, corn and corn products, and cane sugar. We eliminated these from her diet. Now, she was eating strictly organic produce, grass-fed meats, and organic eggs. She added lots of sardines and veggies, plus she ate an avocado every day. This ensured that she would be getting plenty of healthy omega-3 fats, which I knew would help improve her skin.

I also recommended that she take each of these supplements twice a day with food.

- Probiotics: Renew Life Ultimate Flora, 30 billion colony-forming units (CFU)

- 400 IU vitamin E

- 1,000 milligrams vitamin C

- 600 milligrams calcium plus 1,000 IU vitamin D (NOW Foods brands)

- 1,000 milligrams fish oil (NOW Foods Ultra Omega-3)

recent review of nutritional supplements for psoriasis. I recommend getting tested for your level of vitamin D and taking 1,000 to 5,000 IU daily, depending on the results of your test. This needs to be monitored by a doctor, and when you achieve normal levels of D, you can switch to a maintenance dose.[8]

In addition, I recommended that Elaine begin her day with this nutrient-dense smoothie, which is packed with eczema-soothing ingredients.

Elaine's Breakfast Smoothie

1 tablespoon aloe vera juice

8–10 ounces water or more to liquefy ingredients

2 teaspoons flaxseeds

1 teaspoon spirulina or chlorella powder

2 teaspoons chia seeds

Ground red pepper to taste

$\frac{1}{4}$ teaspoon ground cinnamon

$\frac{1}{2}$ cup frozen organic blueberries

$\frac{1}{2}$ organic banana

$\frac{1}{2}$ cup organic kale or spinach

Juice of 1 lemon

1 teaspoon matcha tea

In a strong blender or juicer, combine the aloe vera juice, water, flaxseeds, spirulina or chlorella powder, chia seeds, red pepper, cinnamon, blueberries, banana, kale or spinach, lemon juice, and tea. Blend until liquefied. Serve immediately.

Finally, I recommended to Elaine that she avoid makeup and massage organic coconut oil on the affected skin several times a day.

Recently, Elaine e-mailed me with some very happy news: Her skin has never been clearer, and what's more, she's lost 19 pounds, virtually without trying. She's delighted that she no longer has to cover up or feel embarrassed about the way her skin looks.

Natural Remedies for Irritated Skin

Beyond cleaning up your diet and using recommended supplements, these tips will help you feel more comfortable as your skin becomes healthier.

Become a moisture nut. I advise people with eczema and psoriasis to be sure to liberally and regularly moisturize their skin—but not with any of the commercial and so-called natural skin creams that contain dairy or wheat proteins (hydrolyzed wheat protein), corn syrup, or other corn products (see "How to Find Safer Skin Care Products" on page 189). These can worsen skin problems for many people. Instead, a simple one-ingredient moisturizer I recommend is pure organic coconut oil. Apply it right after a shower while your skin is still slightly damp to lock in the moisture. Generally you will need to apply it only twice a day, in the morning and before bedtime. Some people prefer apricot or avocado oil. Just make sure that you are not allergic to the oil that you use.

Choose organic fabrics and allergen-free laundry soaps. Wear nonitchy, strictly organic fabrics—cotton is best—and wash your clothes in mild, fragrance-free organic laundry soap.

Keep your cool. Hot, sweaty skin aggravates eczema and psoriasis, so stay as dry as you can and shower after you've exercised.[9, 10]

• •

DR. HOWARD'S Q&A

Q. Is there a safe cover-up makeup I can use to hide the awful-looking red patches on my face until they heal?

A. My favorite is jane iredale mineral foundation. I first learned about the iredale products when a friend had some facial resurfacing done and was given the makeup by her doctor, who told her it would be safe for her pretty badly reddened skin. When I first saw her, she had the makeup on, and I didn't even know she had had anything done! But when she took off the makeup, I could see the burn.

Headaches and Migraines

There are headaches, and then there are *headaches*. Common garden-variety headaches trouble almost all of us every now and then. Virtually anything can cause them, including stress, caffeine withdrawal, dehydration, muscle tension, hangovers, and being too tired or too hungry. Most of the time, a plain old headache will quickly disappear all by itself—if we don't chase it away with a couple of pills (such as ibuprofen, acetaminophen, or aspirin) first.

What's That Pain in My Head?

In this chapter, we're not discussing those trifling headaches. I'm talking about chronic headaches painful enough to prompt 45 million Americans to seek medical attention for them. Troublesome headaches of this magnitude are common, and they affect about 38 percent of adults every year.

We call these moderately severe throbbers—which can feel like a band is tightening around your head—tension headaches. They may last anywhere from a half hour or so to several days. Tension-type headaches begin when pain-sensitive nerve endings in your head—for any number of reasons—send impulses to the part of the brain that interprets pain signals from the rest of the body.[1]

Anatomy of a Migraine

And then there are migraines. If you've ever had a migraine headache, you'll know that it's a far more painful vexation than a simple tension headache. Migraines can be preceded by bizarre warning signals, which can include visual disturbances called auras. You may experience tunnel vision, temporary blind spots, seeing stars or zigzag lines, and blurring. You could also have eye pain. These symptoms most often occur about 15 minutes before the onset of the migraine, though they could strike anywhere from a few minutes to 24 hours beforehand—or not at all. Not everyone who gets migraines will experience an aura. Other migraine warning signals can include yawning, difficulty concentrating, nausea, and trouble finding the right words.

Once a migraine develops, you'll know it—the symptoms can be fierce. What may start off as a dull ache can escalate within minutes or hours to severe pain on usually one or sometimes both sides of your head. You may be dizzy or nauseated, and you might even vomit. You could be exquisitely sensitive to light or sound and need to retreat to a dark, quiet room. Some people sweat or feel chills, fatigue, numbness, or weakness, or lose their appetites.

Even after the migraine resolves, you could have lingering symptoms, including neck pain, sleepiness, or feeling a little dull or confused.

We know that some people are sensitive to certain migraine triggers. These include:[2]

- Caffeine withdrawal
- Changes in sleep patterns or too little sleep
- Alcohol
- Stress or physical exercise
- Loud noises or bright lights
- Certain odors
- Missed meals
- Certain foods high in tyramines, like aged cheese or figs

In this chapter, I'll discuss how to deal with chronic headaches as well as migraines. And both relief programs start with your diet.

The No More Pills Headache-Fighting Plan

One key to battling headaches is identifying any delayed-type food allergies you may have because allergic reactions can trigger both tension and migraine headaches. In my experience, getting people off allergenic foods or additives is often all that's needed to alleviate headaches. Dairy, gluten, MSG, aspartame (Equal, NutraSweet), sulfites, and food dyes are prime culprits.

Here is the connection between allergies and migraines: In delayed-type reactions to foods or additives, antibodies attack the foods you've eaten to which you are allergic. This creates highly irritating particles called antigen-antibody complexes. These enter your digestive system and circulate throughout your body, irritating the linings of your gut and blood vessels. Irritated blood vessels become unstable (the medical term is *vascular instability*). The blood vessels contract and expand erratically and can trigger migraines.

Just as certain foods can trigger headaches, other foods can potentially prevent them, or at least dull the pain when they strike.

Wild salmon, sardines, and herring. An international research team, including scientists from the National Institutes of Health, examined the effects of dietary fats on chronic headaches. They learned that eating more omega-3s, which are found in fish, reduced headache pain and improved quality of life for people who suffered from chronic headaches. The study was published in the journal *Pain*.[3]

Vegetables and fruits. The No More Pills Plan focuses on antioxidant-rich vegetables and fruits. For headaches, I don't single out specific varieties for you to enjoy. I want you to eat several servings of multicolored organic produce a day to make sure that you're getting the most complete range of inflammation-fighting antioxidants. Choose the most colorful, freshest (or frozen) produce you can find.

Ginger. This spicy rhizome helps keep blood vessels dilated, which can help prevent migraines. Use fresh or powdered ginger liberally in cooking to enhance most meals. Or use naturally pickled sushi-style ginger (with no artificial color added). As an occasional treat, nibble crystallized ginger candy.[4] Or make ginger tea: Pour boiling water over three thin slices of fresh gingerroot, cover, steep for 10 minutes, and add a few drops of honey.

Headache Trigger Foods

The basic No More Pills Plan is virtually allergen-free, so the perfect place to start when you're dealing with headaches. The plan also bans food additives, which is great for headache sufferers, since many of those chemicals are linked to headaches. According to the National Headache Foundation, the following additives can trigger headaches, particularly migraines, for some people.[5]

- Aspartame
- Nitrates
- Nitrites
- MSG
- Sulfites

Beyond chemicals, I previously mentioned that certain foods, known as high-tyramine foods (even some that may be included on this plan and are fine for people who are not vulnerable to migraines), may trigger headaches in some people. Foods commonly associated with headaches, particularly migraines, include:[6, 7]

- Aged cheeses
- Avocados
- Bananas
- Caffeine
- Chocolate
- Citrus fruit and juices (½ cup a day usually is okay)
- Dried fruit, especially figs
- Peanuts
- Raw onions
- Red wine and red wine vinegar
- Smoked or cured meat
- Sourdough and other heavily yeasted breads
- Soy nuts

Medicating a Migraine?

When you visit your doctor for migraine relief, she's likely to reach into her pharmaceutical toolbox to offer aid. That's not the first approach I'd take. Instead, I'd examine your diet first and eliminate any food allergies. I'd also ask about your home and office environments to see whether you could be allergic to anything surrounding you. I'd work with you on strategies for easing the stress in your life. I might even ask you to keep a headache journal so we could identify potential triggers.

If we ruled out all of your triggers and you still had headaches, I'd probably try traditional Chinese medicine (TCM) to see if rebalancing your system via diet, massage, Chinese herbs, and acupuncture could ease your problem.

I also might use the herbal treatments butterbur or feverfew (see page 198). But if TCM or Western herbs turned out to be ineffective for you, and if your migraines were severe or frequent, I might turn to pharmaceuticals to see if one or more could help you.

My drug choices would be informed, in part, by a 2013 study published in the *Journal of General Internal Medicine*. The researchers found that some FDA-approved medications, including beta-blockers and angiotensin inhibitors, worked better than a placebo and prevented 50 percent or more headaches in 200 to 400 people, per 1,000 treated. Those drugs had fewer side effects than did other drugs that are prescribed off-label for headaches, including antidepressants and anticonvulsants.[8]

Another class of drugs, called triptans, can head off a migraine if you catch it early on. However, they're not for people with known or suspected cardiovascular disease as they may increase the risk of heart attacks or strokes.[9] In my experience, triptans can be especially helpful for menstrual migraines.

Soothing, Natural Headache Treatments

The therapies outlined in Chapter 5 can go a long way to helping ease headaches, particularly tension-type headaches. I also recommend these proven strategies.

Massage. Two kinds of massage have been studied for its effects on migraines with positive results. In a 2006 study, 47 migraine sufferers either were treated with weekly 45-minute massage sessions for 5 weeks or were in a nontreatment control group. The massage was designed to relax muscle tension in the back, shoulders, neck, and head. Those who got the massage had fewer migraines and reported sleeping better, both during the massage trial and for 3 weeks afterward, compared to people in the control group. People who got the massage treatment also had lower heart rates and levels of the stress hormone cortisol. They also reported reductions in their anxiety.[10]

A specific type of massage called craniosacral therapy is a gentle technique during which practitioners relax the soft tissues surrounding the central nervous system. In a small 2012 study, 20 people with migraines had six craniosacral massage treatments over 4 weeks. The researchers gave the participants a test that measures the effectiveness of headache treatments and learned that the therapy significantly lowered headache test scores.[11]

Meditation. In a small pilot study, researchers assigned 19 people with migraine headaches to one of two groups. The first group took an 8-week mindfulness-based stress reduction (MBSR) course that taught meditation and yoga. The other group received standard migraine care. At the end of the study, people in the MBSR group reported having one fewer migraine a month and less severe headaches than did people in the control group. The 2014 study was published in the journal *Headache*.[12]

Pain-Fighting Supplements

These treatments can go a long way to helping you banish headache pain.

Triple therapy. Alexander Mauskop, MD, a neurologist and acupuncturist who's been treating and studying headaches for some 25 years, is the director of the New York Headache Center in New York City. In *What Your Doctor May Not Tell You about Migraines*, his 2001 book, he describes this simple therapy for easing migraines:

- 300 to 400 milligrams magnesium
- 400 milligrams riboflavin
- 100 milligrams feverfew

Dr. Mauskop recommends breaking the dosage in half and taking it twice a day with meals. The formula is also available as Migrelief, available online and at health food stores.[13]

Butterbur. A review of studies that included 293 people with migraines showed that the herb butterbur reduced the frequency of migraine attacks after people took it for 3 to 4 months. Petasin is a compound contained in the plant; it's considered a major anti-inflammatory. "I've had patients get off their migraine prescriptions after taking butterbur," says Aaron Michelfelder, MD, professor of family medicine and bioethics at Chicago's Stritch School of Medicine. The supplement Petadolex contains the extract used in the studies. Follow label directions.[14]

Feverfew. This is a centuries-old European herbal medicine for headaches and many other ills. The migraine-relieving activity of feverfew is likely due to its complex of compounds, including parthenolide; together, they ease inflammation and help relieve smooth muscle spasms. Feverfew also helps prevent the constriction of blood vessels in the brain (one of the leading causes of migraine headaches) and inhibits the production of prostaglandin hormones, which can inflame blood vessels. Finally, feverfew makes platelets "less sticky" and normalizes bloodflow, which may also help reduce migraine frequency and severity.[15] Choose feverfew products standardized to 0.2 to 0.35 parthenolides; the dose is 50 to 100 milligrams daily.[16]

Ginger. In a 2014 study, 100 people with migraines were treated either with 50 milligrams of sumatriptan, a migraine drug, or with 250 milligrams of powdered ginger. Before taking either medication, 22 percent of the people in the sumatriptan group and 20 percent of the people in the

Meredith Mastered Her Migraines

Meredith Richard, 28, of Northfield, Illinois, came to see me recently. She'd suffered migraines since childhood, along with the skin condition eczema. Her doctor prescribed a migraine medication in 2007, but she quit taking it after a year because of its intolerable side effects. She was pregnant when she came in for her first visit with me, and by this time, she was having migraines twice a week, up from her usual frequency of twice a month. Because of her pregnancy, she obviously couldn't take migraine meds even if I thought that was a good option for her, which I didn't.

I tested her for food allergies. She turned out to be reactive to gluten grains, buckwheat, oats, and alcohol and borderline reactive to yeast, pineapple, and avocado. We took her off all of those foods, and, as I suspected they would, her migraines completely vanished. It was wonderful for her to be migraine-free throughout her pregnancy, and especially during those first few months of sleep deprivation in her baby's early infancy.

We also tested some other family members, including her toddler son, who had extremely bad eczema and food-mood issues. Here's what Meredith said about that: "Anyone who was initially skeptical of the allergy testing who then saw the transformation in my son became a true believer. His horrendous eczema and behavior changed just 2 days after we put him on a dairy-free diet."

ginger group reported having severe headaches. Two hours after treatment, 64 percent of the people who'd taken the ginger and 70 percent of the people in the sumatriptan group experienced a 90 percent reduction in headache pain. In the sumatriptan group, 20 percent of people reported side effects that included dizziness, vertigo, and heartburn; 4 percent of people in the ginger group reported mild indigestion.[17] Guess which treatment I'd try first? (Hint: It's not the pill!)

• •

DR. HOWARD'S Q&A

Q. If I follow all of the suggestions in this book and still get the occasional tension headache, what's the safest pain reliever to take?

A. Before you take any medicine, try drinking a full glass of water and doing some relaxation breathing. If that still doesn't work, it's okay to take two acetaminophen.

IBS and GERD

People who have gut problems may be among the most misdiagnosed and poorly treated people when they finally come to my office. And from where I sit, it seems that the number of people who deal with digestive problems is rising sharply. Recent statistics will back me up: As many as 20 percent of adults in this country have some kind of digestive problem.[1]

Trouble in the Gut

Before I define the common problems that affect the digestive system, here's my opinion: I consider most diagnoses of troubled guts to be "garbage" diagnoses. This means that most diagnosticians don't look to the *causes* of these varied gut problems; they simply look at the problems as collections of symptoms. Then they label them as IBS (irritable bowel syndrome) or GERD (gastroesophageal reflux disease) or something else, and they set out to treat the symptoms with drugs or even with invasive procedures.

Those approaches fail all too often because the symptoms, troubling as they may be, aren't actually the problem. The *cause* of the symptoms, most often delayed-type reactions to foods, is the problem, and that's what needs to be treated. Once you eliminate the cause, you'll eliminate the symptoms.

Here's the saddest thing about all of this: A diagnostic code that in most cases is much more accurate than the IBS or GERD label already exists. It is *allergic colitis* and refers to food allergies that cause gut irritation. But sadly, very few physicians ever connect food allergies to their patients' symptoms. There is a ray of hope, however. Finally, specialists in allergies and gastroenterology have recognized the link as FPIES, or food protein–induced enterocolitis syndrome. It becomes official this year (2015). Let's hope medical professionals will now recognize that food allergies can cause irritation to the digestive system. And let's hope that they will begin to use this diagnosis and will treat these conditions by helping people alter their diets. For more information, visit fpiesfoundation.org.

Healing Carla's Constipation

I recently saw Carla Patton, a 66-year-old woman who came in with a life-long history of constipation. She said it started when she was about 5 years old, and she recalled having "every kind of test," including a colonoscopy. She experienced bloating and gas after eating, along with the constipation. She practically lived on the laxative MiraLAX. She followed a gluten-free diet, had oatmeal every morning for breakfast, and ate a generally healthy diet. Still, she couldn't get rid of the constipation.

I tested her and we discovered she was reactive to gluten, buckwheat, oats, food additives and dyes, and red and white wine. She also tested as borderline reactive to peanuts, almonds, cane sugar, corn sugars, and goat's milk. I removed additives, dyes, gluten grains, buckwheat, and oats from her diet and gave her a probiotic.

She came for a follow-up appointment 2 months later and was thrilled that her constipation symptoms had finally vanished. But 2 months later, she called to report she was constipated again. Thinking she was "safe," she had begun including some of the foods containing her "borderline" allergens, so I advised her to stop them. She did, and that resolved her problem.

Many Problems, Many Symptoms

When your gut stops functioning the way it's supposed to (I'll outline the reasons for this a little later), all kinds of problems occur. In the past, doctors diagnosed these functional problems under such conditions as mucous colitis, spastic colon, nervous colon, functional dyspepsia, or spastic bowel.[2]

Various manifestations of IBS include changes in your bowel habits accompanied by abdominal pain, bloating, and cramps. Typically, people dealing with IBS experience constipation or diarrhea to one degree or another. In our current failed diagnostic system, we now divide the "garbage" diagnosis of IBS into smaller "garbage cans." Four IBS subtypes are recognized: IBS with constipation, IBS with diarrhea, mixed IBS, and unsubtyped IBS.

An IBS diagnosis is usually made only after you've been in discomfort for at least 3 months and if you have no other disease or injury that could be causing your symptoms, meaning all tests—blood tests, celiac disease screening, bowel biopsies—have come back as "normal."[3, 4]

When your doctor diagnoses you with IBS, what she's actually doing is telling you what you *don't* have; she is ruling out other types of bowel problems—cancer, infection, or an inflammatory bowel disease such as Crohn's disease or ulcerative colitis.[5] IBS is a rule-out diagnosis that means, "You're sick, and we know it's not cancer or any specific inflammatory bowel disease, but we don't really know why you're having digestive problems."

Your GI Tract

The gastrointestinal (GI) tract, or, more popularly, the gut, is a series of tubelike organs that allow you to digest what you eat and drink; the tubes basically connect your mouth to your anus. Muscles flex and unflex the GI organs, which release hormones and enzymes that act on food and turn it into the nutrients your body can absorb.

The GI organs include your mouth, esophagus, stomach, small intestine, large intestine (including the appendix, cecum, colon, and rectum), and anus.

The No More Pills Plan for Fighting Gastrointestinal Problems

When someone comes in to see me for help with their digestive complaints, I usually start by putting them on an elimination diet to see whether or not they're reacting to any of the foods they commonly eat. Often, the problem is foods containing gluten; other people have problems with dairy, corn, or soy. Many people react to food additives, which is another reason why I urge you to choose organic foods exclusively.

To learn more about elimination diets, see Chapter 2 to get started. Alternately, you could opt for ELISA testing to determine what your triggers might be.

Neutralize What You Eat

The No More Pills Plan is already pretty friendly to people with IBS since it doesn't contain most of the key IBS dietary triggers, which include gluten, dairy products, legumes, additives, and artificial sweeteners. But even some of the healthy foods on the plan may trouble some people with IBS. If you're among them, use this handy guide.[6] Be sure that all fruits and veggies are organic. Lean protein foods—including wild fish and grass-fed beef, pork, and lamb, as well as organic poultry—should be fine for most people with IBS.

Eat these veggies:

Carrots	Spinach
Celery	Squash
Eggplant	Sweet potatoes
Green beans	Zucchini

Limit these veggies:

Artichoke	Leeks
Asparagus	Onions
Brussels sprouts	Shallots

Avoid these veggies:

Broccoli	Cauliflower
Cabbage	Sauerkraut

Eat these fruits:

Bananas	Citrus fruit
Berries	Grapes
Cantaloupe	Kiwifruit

Avoid these fruits:

Apples	Pears
Dried fruit	Watermelon
Fruit juice	

Watch Your Drinking

While you're dealing with IBS, it's important to drink about 64 ounces (or 2 quarts) of pure, filtered water a day. You can substitute green or black tea as well as other unsweetened herbal teas. However, since caffeine can stimulate activity in the colon, which could worsen diarrhea, limit caffeinated beverages or switch to decaffeinated drinks.

Carbonated beverages can also worsen diarrhea—and so can alcohol. Drink no more than one glass of red wine every couple of days; cut back if it causes problems, and, of course, don't drink it if you've tested allergic to wine.[7]

The Stress-Gut-Bacteria Connection

You know the reference to having a "gut feeling" about something? It's not just a clichéd turn of phrase. There is, in fact, a brain situated in our guts. As a matter of fact, there's an entire nervous system down there, called the enteric nervous system, housed within the lining of the digestive tract. It contains neurons that sense when food is moving through the gut, at which point the neurons signal muscle cells to start contracting and pumping the food along, breaking it down into nutrients and waste. During the process, neurotransmitters, such as serotonin, interact with the central nervous system. It's quite a miraculous process.

Even more miraculous is this: Your gut is actually a world of its own, populated by a microbiome of up to 1,000 distinct species of living bacteria and other organisms. A staggering 100 trillion bacteria and other microbes live in your gut—in fact, you contain 10 times more microbes than human cells! And research is revealing the intricate ways in which these microbes interact with our health; immune function, obesity, allergic diseases, and even neuropsychiatric diseases could be linked to changes in the intestinal microbiota. Among the conditions linked to such changes are IBS and inflammatory bowel disease.[8, 9, 10]

Stress can upset your inner world of microbes. When you're under severe stress, your system releases a flood of stress hormones to slow or even stop digestion. That's nature's way of diverting energy to help you deal with the crisis at hand. The stress of an argument at dinner or a postluncheon speaking engagement can also disrupt digestion, leading to cramping or other symptoms. It's entirely possible that stress hormones negatively affect your gut microbe balance and help produce the symptoms that cause so much discomfort.[11, 12]

So it's easy to understand why stress-reduction techniques are high on my list of strategies for dealing with digestive problems. They play an important role in helping you learn to "disconnect" from stressful events and prevent the cascade of stress hormones from flooding your system and triggering the symptoms we call IBS. There's enough science behind each of these approaches to convince me that they're helpful for people with gut problems. Find the approach that resonates best with you.

Cognitive behavioral therapy (CBT). A 3-month study of people with IBS symptoms found that CBT beat simple patient education and improved overall symptoms and well-being, though it didn't relieve pain.

Relaxation therapy. A number of techniques, including restful music, visualization, and progressive muscle relaxation (you consciously relax the muscles in your toes and progress up your body, slowly and systematically relaxing all your muscles moving up your body, until you've relaxed the muscles in your face and head), can help blunt your reactivity to stress.[13]

Hypnotherapy. A form of this practice is called gut-directed hypnotherapy, or GDH, and it's specifically designed for people with IBS and other digestive problems. What's more, GDH might be helpful for people whose symptoms aren't stress-related. In one study, people with severe IBS had 3 months of hypnotherapy treatments. In the treatments, they were directed to place their hands on their bellies while being asked to feel warmth and imagine they had control over their gastrointestinal functioning, reported the *Harvard Health Letter* in 2010. By study's end, participants in the hypnotherapy group reported significant symptom improvement compared with those who were in a supportive psychotherapy group. And in another study, researchers reported that the benefits of gut-directed hypnotherapy could last for years.[14, 15]

Choose IBS-Friendly Supplements

My first step when treating a patient with IBS is to target the cause of the symptoms. Usually, it's a delayed-type allergy to certain food proteins, so I obviously would recommend that the patient banish those foods from her diet. Then, as mentioned, I'd put her on the low-allergen No More Pills Plan. I'd also recommend that she take these supplements.

Probiotics. I list probiotics first because it is absolutely the most important supplement you can take for your gut—and that's confirmed by a 2014 review of more than 40 studies that concluded that taking probiotics eases pain, bloating, and flatulence. Take one capsule a day of a probiotics product that contains 30 billion to 50 billion colony-forming units. Choose a probiotic containing a good mix of organisms, such as my favorite, Renew Life Ultimate Flora. If you have ever had digestive problems, I recommend you take probiotics every day from now on. Interestingly, the latest studies show that the brain has some of the same receptors as the gut and that taking probiotics can even improve brain function, including memory.

Fish oil. Researchers recently discovered that people who have IBS also have deficiencies in their blood levels of long-chain fatty acids; fish oil helps fill that gap.[16] In my book, fish oil is another "take it every day from now on" basic. I like NOW Foods Ultra Omega-3. Take one a day.

Peppermint oil. According to a 2014 review of treatments in the *Journal of Gastroenterology,* enteric-coated peppermint oil is considered a first-line treatment for IBS cramps and pain. Take one or two capsules three times a day between meals.[17]

Curcumin. This phytochemical, responsible for the spice turmeric's brilliant yellow hue, reduced IBS symptoms by 50 percent in a study published in 2004. Curcumin supplements may help by reducing inflammation and abnormal muscle contractions in the bowel. Take 300 to 400 milligrams three times a day with a meal that contains some fat.

Slippery elm. This soothing herb, made from the bark of the slippery elm tree, can heal irritated digestive tract tissues. You can find slippery elm lozenges in health food stores and some drugstores.[18]

Chamomile tea. Delicate chamomile is known for its anti-inflammatory, antispasmodic, tranquilizing, and muscle-relaxing effects, which is why it's a great remedy for IBS pain. Steep one organic teabag in a cup of boiled water, covered, for 10 to 15 minutes. Sip three or four times a day between meals.[19]

Caution: If you know or even suspect that you're allergic to ragweed or if you have hay fever, avoid chamomile. It is in the same plant family as ragweed and often causes reactions in ragweed-allergic people.

GERD: A Gut Problem
Often Linked to IBS

Unfortunately, a number of people with IBS often also suffer from other problems, including chronic fatigue syndrome, chronic pelvic pain, temporomandibular joint disorders, depression, and anxiety.

Gastroesophageal reflux disease (GERD) is also more common among people with IBS than the general population. In this condition, stomach contents flow back up the esophagus, usually due to a weakness in the muscle between the stomach and the esophagus, or that muscle may relax when it's not supposed to.

As I noted earlier in this book, GERD was formerly known as heartburn or acid indigestion, but these days, it's become an official disease, with a host of drugs designed specifically to treat it. GERD is another one of my pet peeve "label diagnoses." You label the problem and find the drug designed to treat it. I've learned over the years that GERD, like IBS, is often triggered by a delayed-type allergy to food proteins. I have had literally hundreds of GERD patients over the years whom I've been able to take off proton pump inhibitors (PPIs) after they made appropriate dietary changes. Now, we're beginning to discover that PPIs have long-term side effects, including the fact that they could interfere with the absorption of key vitamins and minerals.[20]

In some cases, GERD can be a side effect of medications, including asthma drugs, calcium channel blockers, antihistamines, painkillers, sedatives, and antidepressants. Smoking, or being exposed to secondhand smoke, can also trigger GERD.

Though the main, and best-known, symptom of GERD is frequent heartburn, it also causes other less obvious symptoms, including:[21]

- A dry, chronic cough
- Wheezing
- Asthma and even recurrent pneumonia
- Nausea
- Vomiting
- Sore throat, hoarseness, or laryngitis
- Difficulty swallowing
- Chest pain

Beware the Sticky Proteins

The sticky proteins in gluten (wheat, rye, barley, spelt), oats and corn (they have their own type of gluten), and casein (in dairy) are most often the cause of GERD. If you react to them, your immune system attacks them and turns the lining of your gut into an inflammatory mess. It is just as if you were allergic to wool and were constantly wearing a wool sweater. Pretty soon, the healthy skin of your arm would become a red, irritated, and possibly even infected mess.

Once you stopped wearing the sweater and applied a healing balm to your arm, your skin would return to normal pretty quickly. The same principle applies to the lining of your upper gut—the area that is affected by so-called GERD.

Easing Carl's GERD (and Other) Symptoms

I saw Carl,* a man in his fifties, for just two visits 2 years ago. Following his first asthma attack at the age of 15 months, he had had continual asthma attacks until his 10th birthday. Then his asthma abated when he started taking medication. But over the years, he developed GERD, headaches, and dizziness. And his sinusitis was so bad that two specialists had recommended surgery; he'd even lost his sense of smell some 25 years before. He didn't want surgery, which is why he came to see me.

With all of his inflammatory illnesses, I, of course, suspected environmental allergens and delayed-type food allergies. It turns out he was reactive to feathers, gluten, corn, dairy, and bakers' and brewers' yeast. So we put him on a No More Pills Plan diet, and he was diligent about sticking to it. He came back in a month and told me, "I feel like I'm at 9½ on a scale of 10!" He was thrilled to report that his sense of smell had returned. His sinuses were clear most of the time; his reflux was almost nonexistent; and he was down to taking his GERD pills only three times a week.

*Name changed

The solution is simple—and pill-free. Remove the offending foods, apply some good probiotics, and pretty soon the "inner skin" (mucosal lining) of the esophagus and stomach returns to normal. When you use probiotics for the upper gut, take them out of the capsule and swallow them with a spoonful of applesauce. They will start working immediately to soothe your irritated esophagus and stomach. And don't take peppermint, as you might for IBS symptoms. For GERD, it acts as an irritant and relaxes the lower esophageal sphincter, making it easier for reflux to occur.

Losing Susan's GERD and ADD

I saw Susan,* a young woman in her twenties, in 2013. She experienced chronic abdominal pain above her navel and was diagnosed with GERD; her doctor prescribed the GERD medication omeprazole. She'd also been diagnosed with attention deficit disorder (ADD). I couldn't help but notice the dark bags under her young eyes.

It turned out she was allergic to food dyes and gluten. I told her that after 21 days on the No More Pills Plan, she could try tapering off the omeprazole. She came back for a follow-up visit 3 weeks later and told me she was feeling a lot better. She looked it! The bags under her eyes were gone; her stomach pains had vanished; she no longer felt bloated after eating; and she was completely off the omeprazole pills.

And her ADD? She said she was concentrating better and, as a matter of fact, had taken a retest and no longer needed an IEP (individualized education program). She's another perfect example of the many manifestations of the great masquerader food allergy, which shows up in so many different forms. She's living proof that inflammation from food allergies can affect every part of your body, even your brain.

*Name changed

DR. HOWARD'S Q&A

Q. I work with a group of people, and we socialize often at restaurants. How can I be sure to get gluten-free foods prepared safely for me?

A. Do your best to steer the group to a restaurant that has a gluten-free menu. Even some of the chains, like P.F. Chang and Outback Steakhouse, have gluten-free menus. And if you're in doubt, just order grilled fish, meat, or chicken; tell them to avoid any rubs, sauces, or marinades. And get a salad with a squeeze of lemon and some honey (most restaurants have it) for dressing and a baked potato.

Insomnia

So many different elements can conspire to wreck your sleep that it can be tricky to figure out exactly what's keeping you awake. Risk factors include your sex (women are twice as likely to experience insomnia as men) and age (65 percent of people over age 65 have persistent sleep issues). Health problems can interrupt your sleep, too, especially if they are painful, cause breathing problems, or make you urinate frequently during the night. Finally, you might be taking a sleep-robbing pill: Antidepressants, beta-blockers, calcium channel blockers, and some steroid medications all list insomnia as a side effect.[1]

Of course, that's just for starters. There's also your sleeping environment. Is your mattress old and lumpy? Are you allergic to your pillows or bed linens? Or are you allergic to the detergent you use to wash them? Is the temperature in your bedroom too warm or chilly? Does your partner snore or thrash around? Do you have a pet that sleeps with you? Noisy neighborhood? Too much light in the bedroom? I could go on and on. Let's start with the basics.

Exactly What Is Insomnia?

You know what insomnia is: You're likely to say you have it whenever you have trouble falling asleep or when you wake up in the middle of the night and can't get back to sleep. Occasional sleep problems like these are virtually universal (and, unfortunately, inescapable). But when insomnia occurs regularly, then you have the real deal.

Medically speaking, insomnia takes several forms: Sleep experts classify insomnia as *short-term insomnia,* when you've had trouble sleeping for less than 3 months; *chronic insomnia,* which means you lose sleep three or more times a week for 3 or more months; and *other,* which is, well, any sleep problem that doesn't meet the short-term or chronic definition. Then there's *terminal* insomnia, which thankfully doesn't mean what it sounds like; it refers to waking too early and being unable to fall back to sleep.[2, 3]

What Happens When We Sleep

What goes on during all those dark hours of downtime? Since we're not engaged in any activities that keep us busy while we're awake—thinking, talking, listening, moving, reading—you'd assume that our brains must be at rest, too, right? Well, not so much.

Actually, your sleeping brain is a hotbed of activity. During sleep, the brain's neural activity plays a role in maintaining memory, for one thing, which is why a lack of sleep makes you feel groggy and forgetful.

We pass through five sleep phases: stages 1, 2, 3, 4, and REM (rapid eye movement) sleep; each stage has its own function. Most people need 7 to 8 hours of sleep a night to operate at their best.

Getting too little sleep is dangerous. Not only does lack of shut-eye leave us drowsy and unable to properly focus the next day (which could cause accidents), it also dents our memory and even our physical performance. In one study of 15,000 people, researchers found out that getting an average of less than 5 hours of sleep a night over a few years resulted in a decline in memory performance equal to the brain's aging 2 years.[4] During sleep,

3:00 A.M. Wake-Up Call?

If you find yourself waking in the wee hours and having trouble falling back asleep, it could be due to nocturnal hypoglycemia, or low blood sugar. When your blood sugar levels dip while you're asleep, it triggers the release of various hormones, including adrenaline, glucagon, and cortisol, which help bring levels back to normal. But these hormones can also stimulate the brain and wake you up.

To counter nocturnal hypoglycemia, make sure your dinner includes some of the complex carbs listed in this chapter, along with antioxidant-rich foods. Then, snack on a few slices of apple or pear with a handful of almonds or walnuts (or spread the fruit slices with a little almond or cashew butter) an hour or two before bedtime.

waste products from cellular activity are typically swept away; without enough sleep, harmful chemicals could build up and brain cells could begin to malfunction. Sleep may also be the period during which your brain exercises important connections that could otherwise waste away due to a lack of activity.[5]

Insomnia: It Starts with Your Diet

I've had many patients who've had insomnia along with digestive symptoms and headaches. The first thing I do is put them on an individualized allergen-free diet based on the results of an elimination diet or ELISA tests. Once we've worked out what they're reactive to, and eliminate it, almost all of my patients have been able to finally sleep well again.

I particularly remember one person who was reactive to gluten and whose only symptoms were anxiety and insomnia. Once she went gluten-free, she began sleeping better and her anxiety resolved.

If you're wondering how it's possible that reactivity to gluten or to other foods could be related to sleep, let me explain. The first thing you need to know is that 80 to 90 percent of the neurotransmitter serotonin is manufactured in your gut. Serotonin affects mood, appetite, digestion, memory, and sleep—to name just a few.

If your gut is inflamed due to food allergies, it can disrupt your body's production of serotonin, and that will absolutely impact your ability to sleep. Start with the No More Pills Plan and give it at least 3 solid, committed weeks. Meanwhile, tweak your diet by adding sleep-supporting foods and eliminating the sleep-stealers.[6, 7]

Sleep-Friendly Foods

Make some sleep-promoting additions to your diet. With certain smart—and tasty—choices, you could actually eat your way to better sleep!

These lean proteins are rich in tryptophan, which tends to support serotonin levels.

Blue crab	Lobster
Canned tuna	Turkey breast and skin
Chicken breast and skin	

The Pills You *Really* Want to Avoid

Many doctors rely on pharmaceuticals to treat insomnia—but these are pills that I believe you should avoid if at all possible. The side effects associated with these drugs can be devastating.[8]

Zolpidem. In 2013, the FDA released a warning about sleeping pills containing zolpidem, found in Ambien, Ambien CR, Edluar, and Zolpimist. The FDA said that these drugs can impair driving and activities requiring alertness the morning after you take them. People who take insomnia drugs can experience mental impairment even if they feel fully awake. The agency also slashed the recommended dose for these drugs. An even more dangerous zolpidem side effect is sleepwalking. Under zolpidem's influence, people have been known to cook and eat food, wander around outside, and even take a spin in the car while not fully conscious. They retain no memory of their frightening activities the next day.[9, 10]

Benzodiazepines. These tranquilizing drugs, often prescribed for insomnia or anxiety, can increase your risk for developing Alzheimer's disease by 43 to 51 percent, according to a 2014 study of 9,000 people older than 66 who had ever used the drugs. The study was published in the *BMJ*.[11] Benzodiazepines include lorazepam (Ativan), alprazolam (Xanax), temazepam (Restoril), chlordiazepoxide (Librium), and diazepam (Valium), among others.[12]

These complex carbs help stabilize blood sugar levels.

Apples	Sweet potatoes
Pears	Winter squash

These good fats improve serotonin levels.

Almonds	Walnuts
Cashews	(or their nut butters)
Pistachios	

Munch on This Fruit

In a 2011 study, when people ate two kiwifruit an hour before bedtime nightly for 4 weeks, it improved their sleep quality by 42 percent, improved their sleep soundness by 29 percent, and shortened the time it took them to fall asleep by 35 percent, compared with people who didn't get kiwi as a bedtime snack. What's more, people who munched on kiwifruit enjoyed 13 percent more sleep than the control group.[13]

Antioxidant-rich foods, including green leafy veggies, citrus fruit, bananas, and tomatoes, are rich in magnesium and potassium, which help promote relaxation and circulation. In addition, a diet rich in calcium helps keep melatonin at sleep-promoting levels. In particular, calcium-rich foods such as dark, leafy greens, nuts, and seeds maintain your calcium levels, which in turn maintain your melatonin levels.[14]

These soothing beverages help you sleep.

Chamomile tea (unless you're allergic to ragweed)	Passionflower tea

Sleep-wrecking foods. Meat-rich, high-fat diets interfere with sleep. Researchers who looked at nearly 500 women in the Women's Health Initiative recognized that women who reported being sleepiest ate high-fat diets.[15]

Abandon these sleep-killing quaffs.[16, 17, 18, 19]

Alcohol	Caffeine (no coffee or black tea after your morning cup)

Do Some Huffing and Puffing

We've known for years that aerobic exercise plays a role in helping you beat insomnia. That was confirmed in a 2014 Brazilian study, which revealed that aerobic exercise not only improves sleep quality for people with chronic insomnia but also eases depression.

In the study, 21 sedentary middle-aged men and women with chronic insomnia were first tested on a treadmill to make sure they were medically able to participate in the study; then, they walked on treadmills at a pace deemed appropriately aerobic for them by the researchers. The participants walked on the treadmills 3 days a week for 50 minutes each session. Four months later, the researchers retested their sleep patterns. The researchers reported it took the participants 14 minutes less to fall asleep, their sleep time increased by 24 minutes, and their REM sleep time increased by a significant 2.5 percent. The participants reported being 30 percent less depressed, and their overall sleep quality improved by 40 percent. (*Tip:* Perform your exercise in the late afternoon or after work, not right before bedtime.[20])

Add Some "Ohm"

When you're stressed, as I've discussed many times in this book, your body releases a flood of stress hormones, including cortisol and adrenaline. These activate and arouse your system, put your body on high alert, and make you more energetic—which, as bedtime approaches, is the very last thing you want to be. Practicing yoga can calm your arousal response, say Harvard Medical School researchers who studied yoga as an insomnia treatment in 2004.

Twenty participants, all diagnosed with chronic insomnia, learned how to perform a basic, easy hour-long seated yoga routine focusing on breathing and meditation techniques. They were instructed to practice it daily, preferably just before bedtime, for 8 weeks. At the end of the study, the participants reported that their total time awake during the night had dropped by about 50 percent and their sleep quality had improved, as did their total sleep time.[21]

Clean Up Your Sleep Act

These tips can help you sleep better.

- Go to bed and wake up at the same time every day.
- Banish the TV and all electronic devices from the bedroom.
- Make sure your bedroom is dark, quiet, and cool.
- Use foam earplugs and a sleep mask, if necessary.
- Banish disruptive pets from the room if you can.

- Practice a wind-down ritual about 30 minutes before bedtime. Dim the lights, turn off the electronics, listen to soft, calming music, or just sit quietly and practice deep breathing.
- If you must get up in the middle of the night, try not to turn on bright lights—rely on soft night-lights instead.[22]

Choose Sleep-Supporting Supplements

If you've given the No More Pills Plan a 3-week trial and you're getting aerobic exercise but still have sleep problems, give these time-tested natural remedies a try.

- Melatonin, 1 to 3 milligrams 1 hour before bedtime
- L-theanine, 200 milligrams one to three times a day
- Fish oil: one 750-milligram NOW Foods Ultra Omega-3 gelcap, once daily
- Hyland's Calms Forté, a homeopathic remedy, per label directions
- Magnesium, 500 milligrams daily[23]
- Passionflower, tincture, ½ to 1 teaspoon in water 30 minutes before bedtime

Losing the Gluten Calms the Brain

Back in 1982, long before anyone recognized the links between gluten and emotional disturbances, I had already begun to observe the food-mood connection. I saw an 8-month-old baby boy who had suddenly turned from a sweet little baby into a wild man who was irritable, hyperactive, and not sleeping through the night. I thought it might be his diet, since his parents had begun to give him a wider variety of baby foods, including some containing gluten. At that time, I did not have our current testing technology, so I tried an elimination diet. We went back to rice and bananas. It was like magic. The sweet baby was back! We added one new food every 4 days and made it safely through applesauce, chicken, and peas. Then we added sweet potatoes and boom! Wild man showed up again, and wild man also had a rash on his neck. So that was the end of the sweet potatoes, and the end of the wild man, and the end of sleepless nights, both for the little boy and his parents. But his diet remained strictly gluten-free.

Years after this, other physicians became aware of the brain-gluten connection, notably David Perlmutter, MD, author of *Grain Brain*. Dr. Perlmutter is one of the few MDs who truly understand the medical importance of food. He is board certified both in neurology and nutrition, and as far as I know, he is the only physician in the United States to hold both of these certifications. I share his belief that anxiety and insomnia can often be pinned down as reactions to food proteins.

Cut to the mid-'90s. A couple came in so the wife could be tested for her digestive problems. When her results came back, she did have some food allergies. The husband was not so sure he wanted to be tested because all he had was a little anxiety, plus some pretty bad insomnia. He didn't have a single digestive problem, sinus congestion, headaches—just the insomnia and anxiety. I thought back to that little boy and told the husband that I suspected his anxiety and insomnia might actually be from brain irritability caused by inflammation from a food. He agreed to be tested, and he was reactive to gluten. He became very exacting in removing gluten from his diet (much harder 20 years ago than it is now), and his anxiety and insomnia resolved completely. Since then I have seen lots of people whose insomnia and/or anxiety improved or disappeared entirely when they removed allergenic foods from their diets.

• •

DR. HOWARD'S Q&A

Q. My husband's snoring keeps me awake, and sleeping in the guest room is not an option. I don't want to embarrass him, but how can I handle this?

A. Snoring is a possible sign of sleep apnea. If your husband is snoring because he has it, he is not getting enough oxygen at night, and this puts him at risk for many illnesses. Make sure he gets tested. Some services now come to your house, rather than having you go to a sleep lab.

Menopause

A friend of mine who'd recently turned 50 loved enlivening her business meetings with a wisecrack or two. One day, she said that she had to stop joking around. When I asked why, she confessed that something bizarre was happening to her. "Every time I make a joke, my face turns beet red and I break out in an all-over sweat. It's like someone's turned the heat way, way up. It's humiliating, and people are noticing," she said.

I immediately recognized what was going on and knew it had nothing to do with her jokes—or the thermostat. She was having hot flashes.

Since my friend only felt the heat when she was cracking up the conference room, she didn't make the menopause connection. But her experience perfectly illustrates just how quirky menopause symptoms can be. By no means are they a one-size-fits-all proposition, because menstruation symptoms can vary wildly from one woman to another.

Of course, women have been dealing with menopause since the days of Eve. But only in relatively recent history have women been living decades beyond the change, having to live through it and cope. In the past, doctors often dismissed this natural transition. Their thinking was, "It's just a few hot flashes, and menopause doesn't last very long." Even now, at a time when boomer women can easily discuss menopause, there's little mention of accompanying symptoms such as fatigue, arthritic pain, or anxiety—or the feeling of not being your old self (although irritability often gets a nod, as in, "I'm out of estrogen and I've got a gun").

Although I consider menopause a natural transition rather than a medical condition, I do believe in treating the most bothersome symptoms. And the No More Pills Plan is a perfect place to start.

The Age of Medicated Menopause

The prescription estrogen drug Premarin for menopause was introduced in 1942 and became wildly popular with doctors and their patients around 1986. That's when the FDA announced that Premarin (named for the pregnant mare's urine from which it's made)[1] could effectively combat osteoporosis. Unfortunately, we soon discovered that many women who took it were getting endometrial cancer. Lesson learned: Giving estrogen without progesterone causes changes to the lining of the uterus that can lead to endometrial cancer. So progestin was added to Premarin; that drug was called Prempro.

In 2002, researchers published the famous WHI (Women's Health Initiative) study; it included more than 27,000 postmenopausal women between the ages of 50 and 79. In my opinion, and that of other experts, it was a poorly designed study; the average age of the participants was 65. Unbelievably, the researchers took women, most who'd been in menopause for 10 to 15 years, and gave them large doses of hormones, referred to as hormone replacement therapy, or HRT. What a terrible idea! That's like taking a car that has been up on blocks for 15 years, putting bad gasoline in it, and trying to race it. And in this case, the bad gasoline was the synthetic hormones used in the study. Our natural hormones are weak forms of estrogen: estriol, estradiol, and estrone.

Now, consider Premarin and Prempro. Though these synthetic hormones are chemically similar to those in the human body, in HRT, they're not formulated in the same ratio as human hormones are. And, unlike your own hormones, which are secreted directly into the bloodstream, HRT is an oral medication that passes through the digestive system, making a first pass through the liver. Neither Premarin nor Prempro contain our natural weaker estrogens; instead, they're made up of estrone, considered to be the most carcinogenic form of estrogen, plus equilin. Equilin is horse estrogen, which in my opinion has absolutely no business being in a human body in the first place.

The results of the WHI study were startling. Women who took Prempro increased their risk for stroke by 41 percent; their risk of having a heart attack rose by 29 percent; and their risk of developing breast cancer increased by 26 percent. A follow-up study of the women a decade later found that women who took Prempro also had an increase in breast cancer rates, and their cancers tended to be advanced and cause death.

But these statistics were compiled from a group of women who were 10 to 15 years past the appropriate age for receiving hormone therapy. And they were given hormones that were so far removed from a woman's natural hormones that they could not be considered a replacement. Today, we have better hormones. We call them bioidentical because they so closely mimic the hormones that we produce naturally in our bodies. It's worth noting that in the WHI study, even with the synthetic hormones used, many of the younger women benefited from the therapy.

I understand that taking HRT is a choice. For those women whose menopause symptoms are excessive and severe, taking HRT for a few months to a few years right around perimenopause can provide nearly immediate relief. If you do choose to take HRT, I recommend taking the lowest dose possible, since we know that even very low doses will protect your bones and ease your symptoms. Ask your doctor to prescribe hormone therapy in transdermal patch form, rather than as pills, or find a doctor who has experience in prescribing bioidentical hormone therapy.

Cruelty to Horses

In my opinion, the process of making Premarin or Prempro is stomach-turning. According to PETA, the nonprofit animal rights organization, to obtain the hormone-rich urine, pregnant mares are confined in stalls so small they can't turn around. They are hooked up to rubber collection bags, and their drinking water is limited so their urine will contain concentrated amounts of equine estrogen. When their foals are born, the mares are impregnated again. This can go on for as long as 12 years. Foals and the worn-out mares usually end up at slaughterhouses.[2]

My Choice for Menopause: Bioidentical Hormones

In my experience, the better solution for relieving troublesome menopause symptoms is to use bioidentical hormones. These have the same molecular structure as our natural hormones; they are compounded in the same type and proportions as our own hormones; and they are absorbed directly into the bloodstream rather than into the digestive system.

The table below compares how closely the HRT options mimic human estrogen and how they enter your system. The closer, the better—that's my recommendation.

A COMPARISON OF HUMAN ESTROGENS, BIOIDENTICAL ESTROGENS, AND PREMARIN

Estrogen Types	Human Estrogen Approximate %	Bioidentical Tri-Estrogen Approximate %	Bioidentical Bi-Estrogen Approximate %	Premarin—Conjugated Equine Estrogen Approximate %
Estriol	80	80	80	0
Estradiol	10	10	20	40
Estrone	10	10	0	43
Equilin (horse)	0	0	0	17
Route of entry	Directly to bloodstream	Directly to bloodstream (under tongue or on skin)	Directly to bloodstream (under tongue or on skin)	Oral

We usually prescribe bioidentical hormones as creams or sublingual (under the tongue) pills. They are generally safe. I have been prescribing them since 1992 and have had only three patients who did not tolerate them well. However, since the correct dosage is crucial, you have to find a doctor who has experience in prescribing them.

These days, it's pretty easy to find a doctor who prescribes bioidentical HRT. Good questions to ask include:

- How long have you been prescribing bioidentical HRT?
- Were you specifically trained in using bioidentical HRT?
- Do you use creams or sublingual drops or pills?
- Is your compounding pharmacy certified?

The No More Pills Plan for Menopause

The No More Pills Plan is a great way to help you get through "the change" with the fewest possible symptoms—and its benefits are scientifically proven.

In an Australian study of more than 6,000 women, researchers scrutinized the effects of six different diets on menopause symptoms for more than 9 years. At the start of the study, which was published in the *American Journal of Clinical Nutrition*, the women were between 50 and 55 years of age. Forty percent of them experienced night sweats, 54 percent had hot flashes, and 42 percent were symptom-free.

It turns out that the women who most closely followed a vegetable-rich Mediterranean-style diet were about 20 percent less likely to report hot flashes and night sweats than those who didn't stick to the diet. On the other hand, women whose diets were high in fat and sugar were 20 percent *more* likely to develop hot flashes and night sweats.[3]

What about Soy?

I'm not a fan of soy supplements that promise to ease menopause symptoms. However, I do think that eating one serving a day of fermented, organic tofu can be helpful. A famous 1976 study, published in *Family Practice News,* showed that Japanese women had a much lower rate of breast cancer than American women—but when Japanese women came to the United States and adopted our diet, their breast cancer rate became the same as ours. Researchers suggested that the Japanese diet, which is richer in fermented soy foods than a Western diet, was behind the lower cancer rate.

Make sure to choose organic, fermented, non-GMO soy foods, such as:[4]

- Tempeh

- Natto

- Miso

- Pickled tofu

- Tamari (a condiment similar to soy sauce)

Enjoy Menopause-Friendly Produce

Based on the Australian study, researchers said that fruits and vegetables were helpful for relieving menopause symptoms. Some on our list below are especially rich in antioxidants. Others contain phytoestrogens, a weak form of estrogen that occupies the estrogen receptors, potentially lessening symptoms. Make sure to enjoy several servings of these veggies and at least two servings of these fruits every day (organic only).

Vegetables

Asparagus	Cruciferous veggies
Beets	Onions
Bell peppers	Sweet potatoes
Carrots	Tomatoes

Fruits

Apples	Pears
Mangoes	Pineapples
Melons	Strawberries

Additionally, I recommend that you track your food intake for a few days to see if you notice a link between certain items and hot flash frequency. Common triggers are caffeine, alcohol, and spicy foods; if these are problems for you, try avoiding spicy foods and limiting yourself to 200 milligrams of caffeine daily (about two 8-ounce cups of coffee) and three alcoholic drinks per week.

Chill Out Symptoms with These Smart Moves

You can protect yourself against hot flashes by digging into a toolbox of smart strategies. In my experience, these have helped many women sail through the change.

Try black cohosh. A few well-designed studies show that this Native American herb eases hot flashes better than a placebo. I'm not entirely sure why, but there are theories that it could affect opioid receptors in the brain, act as an antioxidant, or have anti-inflammatory properties. The most tested product is Remifemin, available at most drugstores. Follow label directions.[5]

Don't forget to exercise. Exercise is a critical component of the No More Pills Plan, and it's one that's especially crucial for relieving symptoms of menopause. Its benefits include helping prevent weight gain, strengthening bones, and increasing muscle mass. What's more, research tells us that exercise can also reduce menopause symptoms, say researchers from Victoria University in Melbourne, Australia, who published an in-depth investigation of research relating to exercise and menopause in 2014.[6]

Lighten up. Since you'll be changing your eating habits on this plan, losing a little weight will likely be a welcome benefit, especially if you're dealing with hot flashes. In one year-long study, women who lost at least 10 pounds (or 10 percent of their body weight) were 23 percent more likely to experience fewer or no hot flashes, according to researchers funded by Kaiser Permanente. Since fat locks in body heat, and since night sweats and hot flashes are your body's way of cooling you off, shedding a few pounds can help keep you cool and reduce your menopause-related symptoms.

Try hypnosis. Hypnotic relaxation therapy reduced hot flashes and other symptoms by up to 80 percent after 12 weeks, according to a study from Baylor University in Waco, Texas. The researchers theorized that deep relaxation could calm brain regions responsible for heat regulation.[7] What's more, hypnosis could improve memory decline, another frequent menopausal complaint. When the Baylor research team reexamined the data from their earlier study in 2014, they learned that hypnotic relaxation offered additional benefits, including improved sleep and mood. It's entirely possible that improving the sleep of menopausal women could also improve their memory.[8]

Spritz some scents. Clary sage and Roman chamomile essential oils may help balance mood swings, while peppermint can chill hot flashes. To make your own cooling mist (especially helpful for night sweats), mix these ingredients in a 4-ounce dark-glass spray bottle. You can find pure essential oils (choose organic only) online or at health food stores.

3 ounces distilled water

1 ounce witch hazel extract

8 drops each of peppermint, clary sage, and Roman chamomile essential oils

Sip some sage. Sage tea is a time-honored herbal remedy for reducing night sweats and excess perspiration. To brew a cup of this savory tea, pour

1 cup boiling water over 1 tablespoon fresh sage leaves (or 1 teaspoon dried). Steep, covered, for 5 minutes, and then strain. Add a little honey or lemon, if you'd like. Enjoy a cup of the tea two or three times a day.[9]

Don't Neglect Your Bones!

Osteoporosis (bone loss) and menopause can go hand in hand because losing estrogen plays a role in osteoporosis. After menopause, women tend to lose more bone than they build. That's why it's critical to make sure you're getting plenty of calcium (only 11 percent of American women get adequate calcium from their diets), along with other bone-building vitamins and minerals. Here's a plan to follow.[10]

- Magnesium, 400–1,000 mg
- Calcium, 500–1,200 mg
- Vitamin D_3, 800–5,000 IU
- Vitamin C, 1,000–5,000 mg
- Boron, 2–9 mg

- Zinc, 6–50 mg
- Manganese, 1–15 mg
- Copper, 1–2 mg
- Vitamin K, 70–140 mcg
- Beta-carotene, 15 mg

Try Traditional Chinese Medicine

As a trained practitioner of traditional Chinese medicine (TCM), I have case files that are full of menopause success stories. I believe that a combination of acupuncture treatments and specially blended Chinese herbs, adjusted depending on each woman's needs, can offer excellent symptom relief. In fact, acupuncture was just proven effective in a 2014 study published in the journal *Menopause*. Researchers analyzed the results of 12 studies that included 869 women, and they reported that acupuncture significantly reduced hot flash frequency and severity. Acupuncture also was proven to have long-term effects that lasted up to 3 months following treatment.[11]

I also use Chinese herbal formulas with wonderful, evocative names, including Free and Easy Wanderer, Two Immortals, Heavenly Emperor,

My Mother Regained Her Equilibrium— And Personality

I became interested in prescribing hormones because I saw firsthand over many years how much they helped my mother. She went into menopause when she was about 50, as I was graduating from high school. Her symptoms were a disaster. She had always been busy and pretty upbeat. But she developed insomnia, had hot flashes so severe that she soaked through several changes of clothes a day, was irritable at best, and even had suicidal thoughts. It was as if she developed a different personality. Our great old-fashioned family doctor, Dr. Kuhl, said that hormone therapy was probably her best shot at regaining her well-being.

Premarin had been on the market since 1942, so he tried that first. It made my mother so sick that she vomited constantly. Then he tried a new injectable estrogen-testosterone drug called Deladumone. It worked like magic; she was her old self again. She went for injections every 2 weeks, and that was it.

Though Dr. Kuhl tried to taper her off the drug, she'd react with terrible symptoms, so he kept her on it. And when the drug went off the market, he used injectable estradiol cypionate and testosterone cypionate instead. By the time he died, I'd gotten my medical degree, so I continued to prescribe it for her. You should have seen my mother between 65 and 84! She sped around in her blue Buick, driving over the bridge from Iowa to Illinois to play tennis with women half her age. She had strong bones and played a mean game of doubles.

Meanwhile, her book-club contemporaries were collapsing with arthritis and other illnesses. But her oldest sister's story was completely different. My aunt elected not to take hormone therapy. She developed postmenopausal bleeding

Women's Precious, and Mobilize Essence, for example. These need to be prescribed by a qualified TCM practitioner; find one at the National Certification Commission for Acupuncture and Oriental Medicine at nccaom.org.[12]

and had to have a hysterectomy. She gained weight. She was too tired to exercise and became diabetic. Then, she was diagnosed with breast cancer.

Obviously, the stories of these two sisters made a lasting impression on me. My mother, who took hormones, stayed healthy and did not get breast cancer. My aunt, who didn't, suffered multiple disabling illnesses.

The hormones my mother took didn't contain estrone or equilin, and they were injected directly into the bloodstream without entering the digestive system, pretty much like the bioidentical hormones I take, and prescribe, today.

My mother enjoyed her life until she got a sinus infection and was given a pill by her new doctor. He failed to look at her chart and gave her penicillin, to which she was highly allergic. Of course she got sick, so she stopped taking the pills. Several hours after she stopped, she collapsed at home. My father called me, and I went racing out to Iowa to see her. She had gone into septic shock; a "super infection" had developed when she stopped taking the penicillin.

She died 20 years ago. My perfectly healthy, tennis-playing 84-year-old mother—whose own mother lived until the age of 93—died, I believe, years before her time. Because of a pill.

But my mother had 35 years of a fabulous life thanks to a concerned doctor and a good medication—the injectable hormones. And that's what this book is really about—a healthy lifestyle, coupled with wise, discerning use of medications, only when necessary, after we've explored the *causes* for an illness. It is a perfect memorial to her that I am writing this now.

Consider Homeopathy

Homeopathic remedies (available over the counter at health food stores and some pharmacies) can be very effective for some women. Some of the most useful menopause remedies include:

- Sepia (boosts confidence)
- Ferrum Phosphoricum (good for reducing redness)
- Belladonna (an excellent herb for sporadic, rapid hot flashes)
- Sanguinaria Canadensis (counteracts hot flashes on the face, neck, and ears)
- Kali Phosphoricum (eases moodiness and nervous irritability)

If you're interested in trying this 200-year-old therapy to resolve your menopause symptoms, I recommend visiting a homeopath, who will determine an individualized remedy based on your specific symptom pattern and habits. You can find a registered homeopath at homeopathy.org.

DR. HOWARD'S Q&A

Q. I started taking HRT when I was in my fifties. But then I stopped because I was worried about side effects. I'm 64 now. Could taking bioidentical hormones help slow down the aging process I'm experiencing?

A. It's pretty much too late now to start HRT again. If the very flawed WHI study taught us one thing, it's this: If you have never taken HRT or have been off it for a number of years, don't start it in your midsixties! However, Chinese herbal medicine has positive effects for menopause and aging in general. Find a qualified practitioner and try an herbal formula.

Obesity

If you ask me, obesity is the epidemic of this young century, and it's one that will end up hurting exponentially more people than any other plague on the planet. The sad truth is, as a people, we are getting fatter, and it's killing us.

In 2014, Stanford University researchers published statistics from 1988 to 2010, reflecting Americans' changes in obesity, belly fat, physical activity, and caloric intake. The news was grim. Our waists are expanding and our bellies are getting bigger. Incredibly, the number of us who get no leisure time activity has more than doubled—in 1988, 19 percent of American women were inactive; as of 2012, that number skyrocketed to 52 percent.[1]

Here are the stats:

- 68.8 percent of American adults are overweight or obese. That's 7 out of 10.

- 35.7 percent are obese. That's 1 out of 3.

- 6.3 percent are extremely obese. That's 6 out of 100.

- 74 percent of men are overweight or obese. That's 3 out of 4.

Fat is far more than a cosmetic problem. Being overweight is a life-threatening health risk. As the scale climbs, so do your odds for developing type 2 diabetes, heart disease, high blood pressure, nonalcoholic fatty liver disease, stroke, osteoarthritis, and cancers of the breast, colon, uterine lining, and kidney.[2]

What's the Cause?

If you think people get fat because they eat too much and exercise too little, you're only partially right. The unfortunate truth? Part of the reason that we're growing fatter than ever is due to our industrialized food supply. We're eating out of boxes, bags, and cans, rather than from whole, natural foods we were evolved to eat over the millennia. In just the last 100 years or so, an evolutionary nanosecond, we've gone from farm to factory eating. There is simply no way our bodies can adapt fast enough to process the additives in these foods—additives like these:

- Food dyes (made from coal tar)
- Artificial flavorings, MSG, sulfites, and aspartame
- Trans fats that block our absorption and elimination of nutrients at a cellular level by compromising the cell membranes
- Sugar content that is beyond anything in human history
- Brominated vegetable oil in sports drinks (also used as a flame retardant)
- Processed corn products, with their chemical residues and their genetically modified content, in the majority of manufactured foods
- Pesticides, antibiotics, and bovine growth hormone in our milk

Not only is the nutrition processed right out of our mass-produced foods, and the additives put in, but many of the additives actually *make you fatter,* such as artificial sweeteners and colors, emulsifiers, and other non-nutritive ingredients. Experts have named these chemicals *obesogens.*

Obesogens interfere with the way our hormone system works; they mess with our insulin signaling; and they affect the way our fat cells function. And sad to say, these chemicals have been deliberately added to our foods to enhance food production, not to improve our nutrition. Processed foods that are loaded with added sugar, salt, and refined grains also play a role in the obesity epidemic.[3]

Ingredients That Fatten Us

Researchers from the department of medicine at Boston Medical Center published a 2014 report on food additives linked to obesity. Here's a partial list.

- Salt
- Sodium benzoate
- Monosodium glutamate (MSG)
- Autolyzed yeast extract
- Sodium sulfite

- Partially hydrogenated vegetable oil
- High-fructose corn syrup
- Sugar (all forms)

Beyond the chemicals that manufacturers deliberately add to processed foods, when environmental pollutants enter the food chain, they also can act as obesogens that contribute to our obesity crisis. These include:[4]

- Bisphenol A (BPA), found in plastic bottles and canned foods
- Phthalates, found in plastic food packaging
- Organic pollutants and pesticides
- Organophosphates

- Carbamates
- Flame retardants
- Dioxins
- Arsenic
- Cadmium
- Lead
- Antibiotics (from animal feed)

TV Makes You Fat

TV commercials that hawk food products are more than annoying—they can actually make you fat, especially if you're already overweight. It turns out that watching food-related commercials does just what the advertiser intended—they motivate you to eat, according to a 2014 study in the journal *Psychology & Health*.[5]

The No More Pills Plan for Weight Loss

I didn't design the No More Pills Plan to be a weight loss diet. And that's a good thing, because I know that when it comes to weight loss, diets are simply doomed to fail. To lose weight and keep it off, you need a satisfying, delectable eating plan that you can stick with for life, not some roller-coaster plan that you hop on and off.

I designed this plan to be as free of food allergens as possible, because I know that immune reactions to foods are a component in every chronic disease we cover in this book. But the No More Pills Plan is also free of all the kinds of foods that contribute to weight gain: no processed foods, no dairy, no sugar, no grain. And because you'll be eating organic foods, you'll be minimizing your exposure to environmental obesogens.

That said, you can maximize your weight loss on the No More Pills Plan by following a few simple rules.

- Enjoy 3 to 4 ounces of lean protein foods per meal.
- Limit nuts to two or three small servings a day (just enough to fill the hollow of the palm of your hand).
- Eat plenty of green, leafy vegetables. Enjoy these with lemon or organic vinegar and a teaspoon of one of the healthy oils on page 58. Vinegar has actually been proven to lower blood sugar (see page 183 in the Diabetes section).
- Have no more than two servings of low-sugar fruits per day.
- Eat carbohydrate foods only at breakfast and lunch.
- Have three to four cups of green tea a day.
- Spice up your food with a tiny bit of hot pepper. This can help you eat 16 percent fewer calories for the rest of the day, and you'll also feel fuller.
- Celery is the new chip! Cut celery sticks into 2-inch-long pieces, and dip away on salsa or small amounts of guacamole or hummus.[6]

Activity Is Essential

I outlined several exercise plans earlier in this book. If your focus is on losing weight, flip right back to Chapter 4 and get started! Becoming active will ensure your success, and interval exercise is a big key—we know, for example, that interval training can lower blood sugar. Be sure to follow the walking plan as outlined, and after a week or two, increase your pace during the interval portion and extend the "full-out" time by a few minutes each day.

Focus on Destressing

One terrible secret about stress is that it can sabotage even your most committed weight loss plans. Here's why: Whenever you're stressed out (a bad day at the office, a tiff with your spouse, a financial worry), your body responds by releasing hormones. Suddenly, you get a shot of adrenaline so that you can spring into action, and a blast of cortisol prompting you to replenish the energy you haven't actually used. You probably already know that when people take steroids, they want to eat all the time, and they gain weight, especially around the waist. Well, when you're stressed, you're on your own steroids. Result? You feel the urge to eat.

Of course, you're probably not going to grab a celery stick. Instead, you'll want a sweet, salty, or fatty treat because you subconsciously know that eating something like that will release happy-making neurotransmitters that blunt your tension. Try these tactics the next time stress overwhelms you.

Get moving. Harness the power of that adrenaline rush by taking a brisk walk around the block. The exercise will get your blood flowing, and you'll flush that cortisol out of your system. What's more, you'll be burning calories instead of eating or storing them as fat.

Join the slow eating movement. When you're stressed, you tend to eat faster, which usually means you'll eat more food than you need. So just slow down, savor each bite, and pay attention to your feelings of fullness.

Forgo caffeine. Having a couple of cups of coffee when you're under stress raises cortisol levels by as much as 25 percent. Since high cortisol levels continue to promote stress eating, it's a good idea to reach for the decaf the next time you're navigating difficult times. If you do, choose water-processed, not chemically processed, decaf.[7]

Breathing Stress Away

In Chapter 5, I reviewed some easy and extremely effective ways to beat stress. One of the quickest is an easy breathing exercise called the 4-7-8 Breathing Exercise, which was popularized by Andrew Weil, MD, the father of integrative medicine.

You can practice this exercise anywhere, and it takes just a few minutes to learn. Commit it to memory and you'll have a tool to calm you down even in the heat of the most stressful times.

You can do the 4-7-8 in any position, but while you're learning, Dr. Weil recommends that you sit down, keeping your back nice and straight. Place the tip of your tongue against the ridge of tissue behind your upper front teeth, and keep it there in a very relaxed way throughout the exercise. Make sure your tongue is relaxed and not rigid. You will exhale through your mouth around your tongue. If it's easier for you, purse your lips slightly.

1. Exhale completely through your mouth, making a whooshing sound.

2. Close your mouth and inhale quietly through your nose to a mental count of four.

3. Hold your breath while silently counting to seven.

4. Exhale completely through your mouth, making a whooshing sound, to a silent count of eight.

5. This is one breath. Now, inhale again and repeat the cycle three more times for a total of four breaths.[8]

Another of my favorite stress busters is the quick coherence technique developed by Doc Childre of the HeartMath Institute (heartmath.org). It is so simple to do.

Step 1: Heart Focus. Focus your attention on the area around your heart, the area in the center of your chest. If you prefer, the first couple of times you try it, place your hand over the center of your chest to help keep your attention in the heart area.

Step 2: Heart Breathing. Breathe deeply but normally as you imagine your breath coming in and going out through your heart area. Continue breathing with ease until you find a natural inner rhythm that feels good to you.

Step 3: Heart Feeling. As you maintain your heart focus and heart breathing, activate a positive feeling. Recall a positive feeling, a time when you felt good inside, and try to re-experience the feeling. One of the easiest ways to generate a positive, heart-based feeling is to remember a special place you've been to or the love you feel for a close friend or family member or treasured pet. This is the most important step.

The Scary Side of Weight Loss Supplements

First, let me say that when it comes to prescription drugs designed to help you lose weight, I believe that they cause more problems than they solve. Various side effects can range from fecal incontinence to heart problems. None of them actually help you to eat more healthfully. I never recommend taking any of these.

But what about all of those miracle-sounding weight loss supplements you see advertised? Not a fan of those, either, I'm afraid. When you see a headline about an herbal or other kind of supplement linked to illnesses or deaths, you're usually reading about a weight loss product. That's because makers of these products often skirt regulations and use sketchy and sometimes dangerous ingredients in their products.

As far as I'm concerned, the best way to burn off fat is to exercise and stay away from grains, sugars, and dairy fat. I think it's wise to avoid so-called natural weight loss products that promise a quick fix. Fall for the promise of "shed pounds like magic" and you might lose not only your cash but also your liver—possibly even your life.

In a 2013 case involving OxyElite Pro, a fat-burning supplement containing the herb *Rauwolfia canescens*, the FDA notified USPLabs that its product was linked to dozens of cases of nonviral hepatitis and liver failure. Turned out, the product also contained the stimulant DMAA, for which no required safety evidence was presented to the FDA. After receiving the FDA's notification, USPLabs voluntarily destroyed some $22 million worth of product.

"Women are often shocked when they end up in the ER and need urgent care for serious liver problems, especially when we trace the liver damage back to the 'herbal' weight loss pills they were taking," says Herbert L. Bonkovsky, MD, professor of medicine at Carolinas HealthCare System in Charlotte, North Carolina, and the University of North Carolina at Chapel Hill. "They thought they were taking a safe, natural supplement that would magically help them shed pounds. Instead, it damaged their liver and made them deathly ill. Some have required liver transplants or have died."

Even when something innocuous, like green tea, is listed as the main ingredient, shape-shrinking products are bad news. "Read the claims," says Daniel Fabricant, PhD, who is the former director of the FDA's division of dietary supplement programs. "If they seem too good to be true, they probably are."[9]

Coping with Emotional Eating

When you eat because you're sad, tired, angry, stressed, or bored, or when you think you deserve a special treat, you're eating emotionally. It's a problem for some 2.5 million people who eat to control their emotions. If you're among them, you're going to have trouble controlling your weight. I've

Lynette Loses Her Allergies— And 100 Pounds

I saw Lynette* during the first 5 years that I began testing people for food allergies. Her case certainly made me understand that one of the major complications of delayed-type food allergies can be weight gain and that the weight loss "cure" can simply be avoiding the offending foods. Lynette, then in her twenties, had come to me for help.

The first thing I noticed was that she was nearly 100 pounds overweight. She was tall, 5 feet 10 inches, so her maximum weight should have been about 170 pounds. She weighed 265. We talked about what she was eating, and I decided to test her for allergies. When the results came back, we discovered that she was allergic to gluten, dairy, chicken, and eggs. She stopped eating those foods in the spring of 1994. By August, she was down to 188 pounds. By November, without doing anything but avoiding the allergenic foods, she had lost a total of 93 pounds and was down to 172.

I believe Lynette's dramatic weight loss was the result of removing the foods to which she was allergic, because doing so helped reduce her inflammation level. How does that help you lose weight? Let's look at a landmark study cited by Mark Hyman, MD, the eminent functional medicine physician and bestselling author.

The study was published in December 2007 and looked at two groups of

treated many "emotional eaters" in my practice, and I've found there are strategies that can be powerfully effective for helping people blunt the emotional messages that prompt them to eat.

Emotional eating is a challenge, especially here in the United States. Our food culture is so ruled by food marketers that they can be impossible to escape. And eating is at the center of our culture—we have entire cable television channels and network TV shows devoted to the celebration of food—in fact, being a foodie is the latest craze. We've got *Cake Boss, Cupcake Wars, Chopped, Master Chef, Top Chef,* and *Iron Chef America,* to name just a few.

children. The first group was overweight and the second was normal weight. The researchers measured three key factors connected to inflammation in both groups of children. First, they measured high-sensitivity C-reactive protein (CRP), a marker that shows the general level of inflammation in the body. Then they conducted ultrasound tests to measure plaque in the carotid arteries (the main arteries that supply the brain). Finally, they tested the children for delayed-type food allergies.

Here's what they found: The overweight kids had three times the level of CRP and had much thicker carotid arteries, which signal early atherosclerosis and heart disease. They also had higher rates of food allergies, which the researchers linked to the inflammation and obesity. As they explained in the study, inflammation from any cause can lead to insulin resistance and higher insulin levels. Because insulin is a fat-storage hormone, when levels are consistently high, you end up storing more fat—particularly around the belly.

Lynette's experience dramatically illustrated what I believe: Eliminating the foods that cause delayed-type food allergies is an effective strategy for treating obesity. You don't even have to limit calories—just the foods to which you're allergic.

*Name changed

So, you're surrounded. Now, how to stop?

First, if emotional eating is really an out-of-control issue for you, you won't respond to the traditional advice, such as: Eat according to your nutritional needs, make your own decisions about food, disconnect food from emotional triggers, eat mindfully, and keep triggering foods out of the house. None of that is going to do you a bit of good.

You have to treat your emotional eating like an addiction—because it is! If it were a matter of being able to talk or discipline yourself out of it, you would have done that already. But, as a wise person once said to me, "You can't 'logic' someone out of something they weren't 'logic-ed' into."

I follow the principles of traditional Chinese medicine when it comes to emotional eating; I focus on the root of the problem, not its symptoms. And the root here is emotions, emotional triggers, and past unresolved emotional trauma. I have seen people who ate to fill up the hole of rejection from their parents. I have had clients who ate to calm the trauma from abuse and who kept eating in a subconscious belief that fat could be their shield against being abused again. I have seen people who were given

Are You an Emotional Eater?

Here are seven signs of emotional eating:

1. You eat when you are actually full, or you think about food when you are full.

2. You eat when you are bored or tired.

3. You eat when you have either negative or positive emotions— when you are angry, sad, disappointed, anxious, or happy—and you describe food with emotional words like decadent or sinful.

4. You eat when you are stressed about getting something done for work or school. You gather your food and then sit there and munch it absentmindedly while you work, almost without even realizing it. And surprise, all of a sudden the big bowl of chips or candy is gone.

5. You have food cravings.

6. You can't stop yourself from eating even if you want to. You binge eat. You are out of control.

7. You eat food to feel good and use it as a substitute for love, comfort, and security.

If two of these describe you, you have an issue with emotional eating. If three describe you, consider addressing your problem, and if four or more describe you, you may want to get some assistance.

When You Need More Help

Research is proving that bariatric surgery can be the most effective way to treat obesity and may even cure type 2 diabetes. In fact, if you're obese, it could reduce your risk of developing diabetes by up to 80 percent, according to a 2014 study funded by the UK National Institute for Health Research.[10] On the plus side, having the surgery gives you an excellent chance of being able to reduce and even stop taking many of the medications you're now on for diabetes, high blood pressure, and high cholesterol. On the downside, you face the side effects that come with any surgical procedure, and you'll have to learn to eat in a completely different way. Following surgery, you'll only be able to eat tiny portions of food. All in all, I do think this is something to consider for the person who is obese and has tried and failed at diet after diet.

food instead of attention as children and now use food as a way of giving themselves love and attention. And, of course, I have seen anorexia and bulimia.

I've found the following strategies help even deeply rooted cases of emotional eating.

Emotional freedom technique (EFT). I described this easy and surprisingly effective therapy in-depth in Chapter 5 on page 106. It's especially good for emotional eating because it helps you deal with past trauma, which in my experience can often trigger emotional eating. EFT relies on bringing your unhealthy old beliefs or habits about food that you took on as a child to the front of your mind, as you tap acupressure patterns on key acupuncture points. Doing so actually changes your habitual neurological pattern. Many people find that working with a trained EFT coach in the beginning is extremely helpful; many do online sessions via Skype. Find a coach and learn more at eftuniverse.com or naturallythinyou.com.

Overeaters Anonymous (OA). If your eating truly feels like an addiction, you could try Overeaters Anonymous, a 12-step program modeled on Alcoholics Anonymous. In OA, you follow a food plan and use the group support and the 12-step methods to keep you on track. I have seen it work well for quite a few people, and it is widely available and free.

Cognitive behavioral therapy (CBT). Cognitive behavioral therapy is an individual short-term talk therapy that aims to change your unhelpful behaviors. The therapy focuses on changing patterns of thought and action in a way that allows you to reach your goals.

● ●

DR. HOWARD'S Q&A

Q. In your opinion, how obese does a person have to be to consider bariatric surgery?

A. Rather than hazard an opinion, I looked up the guidelines. Here they are, from the Cleveland Clinic.

Research supports the benefits of weight loss surgery for those with a body mass index (BMI) between 35 and 39.9 and obesity-related health conditions, such as type 2 diabetes, obstructive sleep apnea, high blood pressure, osteoarthritis, and other obesity-related conditions. You could be a candidate for surgical weight loss if you meet any of the following criteria:

- You are more than 100 pounds over your ideal body weight.

- You have a BMI of more than 40.

- You have a BMI of more than 35 and are experiencing severe negative health effects, such as high blood pressure or diabetes, related to being severely overweight.

- You are unable to achieve a healthy body weight for a sustained period of time, even through medically supervised dieting.

Sinusitis

When you're struck with sinusitis, your face can feel like a punching bag. Your cheekbones hurt, your eyes hurt—even your eyebrows ache. Blame it on your poor sinuses. You'd probably been coping with allergies or a cold, which eventually inflamed these air-filled spaces around your nose, eyes, and cheeks. Now your sinuses are infected and congested. And you're too weak to fight back because you may also have a fever, all-over body aches, and bone-melting fatigue. Sinusitis, which medically speaking means sinus inflammation, is bad enough—but if your sinuses become infected, you're in for a nasty, lingering problem.[1]

Four kinds of sinusitis exist:

- Acute: lasts up to 4 weeks
- Subacute: lasts from 4 to 12 weeks
- Chronic: lasts for more than 12 weeks and may continue even for years
- Recurrent: when you have several attacks in one year

The No More Pills Environmental Clean-Up Plan for Sinusitis

One of the really rewarding aspects of this No More Pills environmental plan is the way it can almost immediately turn around a condition like sinusitis. That's because the symptoms of food allergies often entail congestion—a runny nose and other upper respiratory problems. If you continually eat the foods to which you're allergic, you could easily become one of those people who gets sinus infection after sinus infection. Remove the foods and environmental offenders, and suddenly the congestion resolves and your sinus problems fade away.

The very first thing I do when someone comes to see me with sinusitis is help them figure out what foods or environmental items could be causing a delayed-type food allergy. I recommend testing for food triggers and also to see whether the patient is allergic to anything in her immediate environment—including pets, feather pillows, furniture, carpeting, even laundry detergent. Once we've identified the triggers, we eliminate them, and very often, that's the end of a person's sinus problems.

Removing just one or two offending environmental items can be almost unbelievably effective. For example, consider the amount of time you spend in your bed. For most people, it's somewhere between a quarter and a third of their lives. But if you're allergic to feathers and house dust, and you're spending that much time head down or even face down on a feather pillow that has collected months to years of dust mites, then it's no wonder you're congested.

Beware Airborne Allergens

If you're allergic to common outdoor allergens, such as tree, grass, or weed pollens or to mold spores, it's wise to limit your outdoor time during the worst of the season. Also, make sure that pollens and mold spores are not circulating in your indoor air by keeping the windows closed and using the air-conditioning—making sure to change the filter in your air conditioner frequently.

At the 2011 meeting of the Healthcare Associated Infections Advisory Committee in London, a research report found that in just 2 years of use, one-third of a pillow's weight is made up of (ugh!) dead skin cells, bugs, dead dust mites, and their droppings. Now, suppose that besides the irritation you'll experience being exposed to all those yucky dead bugs, dust, and debris, you're also allergic to dust mites and feathers. Get rid of that old pillow, and voilà! You'll be able to say goodbye to a major portion of your sinus problems—if not all of them—in one fell swoop. I counsel my allergic patients to get down-alternative pillows and to put dust-barrier pillow covers on them and on the mattress.

What's more, your bedroom carpet may be the "monster under your bed." It's best not to have carpet in the bedroom. If you do, treat it every 6 months with the dry carpet cleaner Capture. You just spread it on the carpet and vacuum it up to keep the nasty little dust mites from taking hold. In studies conducted at Johns Hopkins University in Baltimore, Capture tested 70 percent more effective at removing allergens than vacuuming alone.

The No More Pills Plan for Clearing Your Sinuses

By now you know that this plan is essentially an allergen-free way of eating. Still, some foods possess extra anti-inflammatory power, which is why I recommend that you focus on serving plenty of these foods, below, that are known to chill inflammation.

- Wild salmon, black cod (sablefish), sardines, and herring
- Tart cherries
- Avocados
- Organic eggs
- Dark, leafy greens
- Green tea
- Pineapple
- Berries
- Spices: ginger, basil, turmeric, red pepper, and horseradish

And even though they're included in the main plan, avoid these foods when you have sinusitis.[2, 3]

- Mushrooms
- Pickled foods
- Wine

Other Treatments for Sinusitis

Most primary care doctors have a stock response for treating sinusitis that includes antibiotics to treat the infection, steroid inhalers to reduce inflammation, and antihistamines or decongestants to help dry up the congestion.

I will occasionally prescribe antibiotics for people when I believe that a bacterial infection is raging, although even then, I may choose traditional Chinese medicine herbal formulas instead. One thing I won't do is prescribe antibiotics for a bad cold. Not only are they useless against colds, they're also harmful. They're useless because colds are caused by viruses, and antibiotics don't kill viruses; they're harmful because of their side effects and because they add to our universal antibiotic-resistance crisis.

But I'm unlikely to recommend the other drugs often prescribed for sinus problems. I don't believe that they're called for, in most cases, and I'm

(continued on page 248)

Mary: No More Tranquilizers

Mary first came to see me in June 2001. The then 44-year-old designer had a punishing schedule and cared for two young children; one was autistic. That child often woke around 2:00 a.m. and stayed up until 7:00 a.m. Mary started her day between 6:30 and 7:30 a.m. so she could get her kids to school, and then she'd come home, where she did her design work.

Her work was a challenge: She needed 30 hours a week to finish her work, and she had a 4-hour window to get it done while the kids were at school. She worked nights and weekends to complete her assignments. The time after school was packed with therapy appointments 5 days a week for her autistic child, and lessons and sports for her other child.

Time for her own care or to de-stress was limited, to say the least. But Mary was resourceful. She hired a babysitter one night a week, and she and her husband traded off being with the kids so that they could each go to yoga or the gym once a week.

Mary's physical problems included congestion and chronic allergic sinusitis. She had known allergies to mold and cats, and she used air conditioning and an air filter in her bedroom. She wanted to get off antihistamines because they made her feel tired, and she just couldn't afford that with her schedule.

I put her on a mold-free diet, gave her homeopathic drops for the congestion, did some acupuncture to clear her sinuses and lower her stress, gave her a Chinese herbal formula, and sent her to be tested for food allergies.

The tests showed that she was allergic to dairy, eggs, and wheat. She came back for a follow-up visit in November, and we discussed ways to manage her allergen-free diet. I gave her enzymes and probiotics to take with each meal. She said she felt a lot better on the diet, and she stopped taking the antihistamines.

I didn't see her again until April 2007. She hadn't stuck with the allergen-free diet; she had edged back to a "normal" diet because her life was so stressed and busy. Also, she had recently broken out in hives from head to toe. She was still eating wheat—a piece of toast every morning—and I also suspected she had become allergic to more foods. I was right. Testing revealed she now had allergies to food dyes, dust, mold, and the following foods: gluten, dairy, eggs (her previous allergies), plus corn, oats, cane sugar, and coffee. I gave her some acupuncture and Chinese herbs to calm the hives and cautioned her to strictly avoid all of her allergens.

She came for a follow-up visit 1 month later. She was working hard on her diet and told me that she'd figured out an additional cause for her hives. She'd been spending time in the house of a friend who had cats, in a space with a hyperbaric oxygen chamber that they both thought was free of cat hair. But apparently Kitty had been using the chamber as a playroom! At that visit, we also did more testing and found allergies to citrus, guar gum, sunflower seeds, and chickpeas.

She visited again in October that year, saying that now her worst problem was fatigue. She'd stuck to her diet and stayed away from the cat, and as a result, her hives had disappeared entirely in September. She'd lost 25 pounds and felt great about that. Her diet was:

Breakfast: Rice cereal or fruit and rice toast
Lunch: Large salad with chicken
Dinner: Meat or chicken, vegetables, potato
Snacks: Raw cashews or fruit

We discussed ways to increase her calorie intake a little bit so that she would not lose any more weight, and I gave her an adrenal supplement for her fatigue.

She came for one more follow-up visit a few weeks later. Her sinus congestion had improved dramatically, and she was feeling much less tired.

I didn't see her again until almost 7 years later, in March 2014. Her now 19-year-old autistic child still needed plenty of her time, but her other child had

(continued)

graduated from college and was home helping out. Now Mary was taking the tranquilizer Klonopin for her stress, which she wanted to stop, and she was also in menopause. Her muscles were tight and sore, despite weekly chiropractic treatments and massage. I suggested we try an emotional freedom technique (EFT) session for her stress. We did one session and I referred her to an EFT practitioner for more. I also gave her an herbal formula for menopause. Additionally, I recommended a Paleo-style diet, very close to what we have on the No More Pills Plan.

She came back to me in April and said that she was doing regular EFT sessions and that it eased her stress from caring for her son. But Klonopin caused unwanted side effects, and her menopausal symptoms had worsened—hot flashes, night sweats, and insomnia. I gave her a prescription for bioidentical hormone replacement therapy, and we talked about how to taper off the Klonopin.

We talked on the phone in September 2014, and it was all good news. She was off the Klonopin; her menopause symptoms had resolved; and she was feeling generally well, able to manage, and, at last, really enjoying life— and taking no more pills!

---

not happy with their side effects. As I've said, once you've removed allergenic foods and environmental triggers, sinusitis symptoms are likely to fade away on their own.

Natural Sinus Support

You may not be able to eliminate all of your symptoms, even after removing allergens from your diet and environment—after all, it's a big world out there, and you don't want to live in a bubble. But these natural treatments can help provide relief for even stubborn sinus problems.

Harness a healing army. Probiotics are "good" bacteria that help strengthen your immunity and shield you against allergies. My favorite brand is Renew Life Ultimate Flora. It's available in several strengths, from 2 billion to 200 billion organisms in each capsule. For most people, I recommend either 30 billion or 50 billion organisms. Take one every day.

Use Boiron Optique 1 eye drops. For me, and many of my patients, these homeopathic allergy drops are amazingly effective. The drops soothe your eyes and the rest of your head as well. They come in individual sterile drop dispensers with a twist-off top. I started taking them four times a day during a peak allergy season, and now I generally take them twice a day, about three times a week, year-round. I have actually felt my sinuses open and clear after using them.

Find Clear Sinus and Ear. This is a combined Chinese herb and homeo-pathic formula that is very effective. I have used this and recommended it to many patients. Find it online, and follow label directions.

Decongest with D-Hist. This product contains a blend of herbal and other ingredients—all of which have good research behind them for their effectiveness against sinus problems—including quercetin, nettles, brome-lain, and the amino acid NAC (N-acetyl-L-cysteine). It's available online; follow label directions.

Try Sinupret. This is a combination European herbal medication that's been clinically tested and proven effective for treating sinus conditions; it

Ban These Sinus-Cloggers

In addition to dust and mold, many household items can irritate your sinuses and clog up your head, including:

- Body products
- Cleaning products
- Fabric softener (liquid or sheets)
- Fire-retardant chemicals on furniture
- Formaldehyde preservatives in carpet or curtains
- Furniture and rug "deodorizing" sprays
- Furniture polish
- Kerosene lamps
- Laundry and dish detergents
- Paint or varnish
- Plug-in or other air "fresheners"
- Scented candles

is also a natural antibiotic. It contains the herbs cowslip, yellow gentian, black elderberry, common sorrel, and vervain. Combined, these herbs clear congestion, ease inflammation, and are natural antibiotics. Find it in health food stores and online. Follow label directions.[4, 5, 6, 7]

Take a steam. Eucalyptus essential oil is a time-honored traditional remedy for helping ease congestion. I recommend shaking several drops of the oil onto a damp washcloth, placing it on the floor of a shower, and then turning on the water as hot as you can stand it. Inhale the steam for 10 minutes or so, and then dry off in a warm room so you don't get chilled.

Robert Recovered from His Sinus Woes

Robert* first came to see me in 2005. He had recurrent sinus infections and congestion. After testing, we learned that he was allergic to tree pollens, gluten, peanuts, and coffee. He was careful about following his new gluten-free diet and did his best to avoid tree pollens. It worked! His sinus congestion vanished.

But recently, I heard from him again. He called to say he had another sinus infection. Because it had become a full-blown infection, I prescribed an antibiotic, and it solved his sinus problems for a while. I gave him a refill so he could take the antibiotics right away if he developed another infection. But when he needed a third round of antibiotics a few months later, I called a time-out.

Pills were obviously not the answer for Robert. We had to figure out what else was going on with him. I asked him to come in to get tested again. It turned out that he was now allergic to feathers, dust, and mold, along with the tree pollens. And he admitted that he'd been eating a little gluten, to which he was still allergic; on top of that, he'd also become reactive to buckwheat, oats, and dairy. (He enjoyed a regular oat-based breakfast bar.)

DR. HOWARD'S Q&A

Q. When I get a bad sinus infection with a fever, should I rest in bed or is it okay to go to work?

A. Stay in bed! Going to work with a bad infection and a fever stresses your whole system and lengthens your recovery. It also puts your coworkers at risk of catching what you have.

Further, he was renovating his Michigan cottage, which was full of dust and mold. As if that wasn't enough, he was also riding his bike in a wooded area that had a lot of soil molds. It was a perfect storm of breathing and eating sinus-clogging stuff—pollens, dust, molds, gluten, oats, and dairy. No wonder the pills didn't work. Poor Robert was lucky to be breathing!

Here was the plan for Robert:

1. Wear a filter mask when biking.
2. Wear a filter mask during cottage rehab.
3. Continue to avoid peanuts and coffee.
4. Strictly avoid gluten grains, buckwheat, oats, and grain-based alcohols.
5. Strictly avoid dairy.

It worked! Just several weeks after he embarked on my five-point plan, his sinus congestion and infections cleared up. And as long as he follows his plan and stays away from his allergens, Robert will no longer be a sinusitis sufferer.

*Name changed

Part III

Recipes

Note: Whenever possible, all ingredients should be labeled USDA organic, especially produce, meat, and poultry. Also, read labels to make sure all ingredients are gluten-free.

Breakfasts

Blueberry Flaxseed Muffins

Makes 6

¾ cup almond meal or almond flour

⅓ cup ground flaxseed

½ teaspoon ground cardamom or 1 teaspoon ground cinnamon

1 teaspoon baking powder

2 eggs

¼ cup honey

¼ cup unsweetened almond milk

1 tablespoon olive oil

1 tablespoon vanilla extract

½ cup fresh blueberries

1. Preheat the oven to 350°F. Coat a nonstick 6-cup muffin pan with cooking spray or line with paper or foil liners.

2. In a medium bowl, whisk together the almond meal or flour, flaxseed, cardamom or cinnamon, and baking powder.

3. In another medium bowl, whisk together the eggs, honey, almond milk, oil, and vanilla. Stir in the blueberries and the flour mixture.

4. Divide the batter among the muffin cups.

5. Bake for 18 minutes, or until a wooden pick inserted into the center of a muffin comes out clean.

Per muffin: 219 calories, 7 g protein, 19 g carbohydrates, 14 g total fat, 1 g saturated fat, 3 g fiber, 129 mg sodium

Turkey and Fennel Breakfast Sausage

Makes 10 servings

1 small carrot, finely chopped

1 rib celery, finely chopped

1 small onion

1 teaspoon coconut oil

1 clove garlic

1 teaspoon fennel seeds

½ teaspoon fenugreek seeds or ground fenugreek

½ teaspoon black peppercorns, freshly ground

½ teaspoon dried basil

¼ teaspoon Himalayan salt

½ teaspoon dried thyme

½ cup ground walnuts

1 pound lean, organic ground turkey

1 egg, beaten

1. Preheat the oven to 350°F. Finely chop half of the onion (reserve the other half). In a medium skillet over medium heat, heat the oil. Cook the chopped vegetables until lightly browned. Be sure not to let the oil smoke. Allow the vegetables to cool.

2. In a food processor, combine the remaining onion and the garlic. Process until finely chopped. Add the cooked vegetables and pulse. Transfer the vegetable mixture to a large bowl and add the fennel seeds, fenugreek, pepper, basil, salt, thyme, and walnuts. Combine until mixed. Add the turkey and egg and mix together until the vegetables and seasonings are evenly distributed.

3. Cut parchment paper into 1 piece approximately 10" long. Place the turkey mixture in the center of the parchment and shape into a large log. Tightly wrap the parchment around the log and place in a baking pan.

4. Bake for 1 hour. Allow to cool and then refrigerate for at least 1 hour. Remove the parchment from the turkey log and slice into 1" disks. If freezing, lay the disks out on a baking sheet and place in the freezer. Once frozen, place the sausage patties into freezer bags and keep frozen until using.

5. In a large skillet, fry the sausage patties until lightly browned on both sides.

Per serving: 125 calories, 11 g protein, 7 g carbohydrates, 7 g total fat, 2 g saturated fat, 1 g fiber, 66 mg sodium

Eggs Florentine

Makes 2 servings

4 eggs

2 teaspoons olive oil

1 bag (6 ounces) fresh
  baby spinach

$\frac{1}{8}$ teaspoon salt

$\frac{1}{8}$ teaspoon ground
  black pepper

1. Preheat the oven to 350°F.

2. Coat four 1-cup custard cups with cooking spray and add 1 tablespoon of water to each cup. Break 1 egg into each cup. Bake for 15 to 20 minutes.

3. Meanwhile, in a small nonstick skillet over medium heat, heat the oil. Cook the spinach, stirring constantly, until wilted. Season with the salt and pepper.

4. Divide the spinach between 2 plates. Place 2 baked eggs on top of each serving of spinach.

Per serving: 273 calories, 15 g protein, 6 g carbohydrates, 14 g total fat, 4 g saturated fat, 2 g fiber, 378 mg sodium

Western Scramble

Makes 4 servings

1 sweet potato (6–8 ounces total weight), peeled and cut into ½" chunks

1 tablespoon sunflower oil

1 onion, coarsely chopped

1 red bell pepper, coarsely chopped

1 green bell pepper, coarsely chopped

½ cup chopped extra-lean organic cooked ham

6 large eggs

½ teaspoon coarsely ground black pepper

Pinch of salt

1. Place the potato chunks in a medium saucepan. Add cold water to just cover. Bring to a boil over high heat. Reduce the heat to a simmer, partially cover, and cook for 10 minutes, or until tender. Drain and set aside.

2. In a large nonstick skillet over medium-high heat, heat the oil. Cook the onion and bell peppers, stirring often, for 8 minutes, or until tender and lightly golden. Stir in the ham and potato chunks and cook, stirring often, for 2 minutes, or until just starting to brown.

3. Meanwhile, in a medium bowl, beat the eggs. Add the black pepper and salt.

4. Pour the egg mixture into the skillet. Reduce the heat and cook, turning often with a nylon spatula, for 3 to 5 minutes, or until just set.

Per serving: 214 calories, 14 g protein, 14 g carbohydrates, 11 g total fat, 3 g saturated fat, 3 g fiber, 263 mg sodium

Honey-Sweet Broiled Grapefruit Halves

Makes 4 servings

2 **medium red or pink grapefruit (about 1 pound each), halved and sectioned**

4 **teaspoons honey**

¼ **teaspoon ground cinnamon**

¼ **teaspoon ground cardamom**

1. Preheat the broiler. Line the bottom of a broiler pan with foil.

2. Place the grapefruit halves in the pan. Drizzle 1 teaspoon of the honey over each half, spreading it evenly. Sprinkle each grapefruit half with a tiny bit of the cinnamon and cardamom.

3. Broil 4" to 5" from the heat for 5 to 7 minutes, or until glazed and heated through.

Per serving: 75 calories, 1 g protein, 19 g carbohydrates, 0 g total fat, 0 g saturated fat, 2 g fiber, 0 mg sodium

Omelet Italian-Style

Makes 1 serving

2 tablespoons chopped
  onion

2 tablespoons chopped
  green bell pepper

2 tablespoons chopped
  tomato + additional for
  garnish

3 eggs, beaten

$\frac{1}{2}$ teaspoon dried oregano

1 teaspoon chopped fresh
  parsley

Heat a medium nonstick skillet coated with cooking spray over medium heat. Add the onion and pepper and cook, stirring occasionally, for 2 minutes, or until sizzling. Add the tomato. Cook for 1 minute, or until just starting to soften. Add the eggs and sprinkle with the oregano. Cook, lifting the cooked edges of the egg mixture with a fork so the uncooked egg can run underneath, for 5 minutes, or until the bottom is set. Cook undisturbed for 1 to 2 minutes, or until the eggs are completely set. Sprinkle with the parsley and fold the omelet in half. Slide onto a plate and garnish with additional tomato.

Per serving: 232 calories, 20 g protein, 5 g carbohydrates, 14 g total fat, 5 g saturated fat, 1 g fiber, 507 mg sodium

Peachy Quinoa Breakfast

Makes 1 serving

⅔ cup water

¼ cup quinoa

1 teaspoon honey

¼ cup sliced fresh or frozen and thawed peaches

2 tablespoons sliced almonds

1 tablespoon unsweetened coconut

Pinch of ground cinnamon

Pinch of ground ginger

In a microwaveable bowl, combine the water, quinoa, and honey. Stir to mix well. Microwave on high power for 2 to 3 minutes, checking after each 30 seconds, or until thickened and the liquid is absorbed. Stir in the peaches and top with the almonds and coconut. Sprinkle with the cinnamon and ginger.

Per serving: 294 calories, 9 g protein, 41 g carbohydrates, 12 g total fat, 4 g saturated fat, 6 g fiber, 11 mg sodium

Super Strawberry Smoothie

Makes 1 serving

1 cup sliced strawberries

¼ cup coconut milk

½ cup vanilla almond milk

¼ cup unsweetened pomegranate juice

In a blender or food processor, combine the strawberries, coconut milk, almond milk, and juice. Blend or process until thick and smooth. Pour into a glass and serve.

Per serving: 218 calories, 3 g protein, 24 g carbohydrates, 14 g total fat, 11 g saturated fat, 5 g fiber, 105 mg sodium

Sweet Potato Pancakes

Makes 2 servings

1 large sweet potato, peeled and cubed

2 scallions, chopped

2 egg whites

⅛ teaspoon ground black pepper

Pinch of grated nutmeg

Pinch of ground ginger

1 tablespoon sunflower oil, divided

1 cup unsweetened applesauce

2 teaspoons maple syrup

1. In a steamer set in a pan of boiling water, steam the potato for 12 to 15 minutes, or until very tender. Transfer to a large bowl and mash until almost smooth. Add the scallions, egg whites, pepper, nutmeg, and ginger and mash to combine.

2. In a large nonstick skillet coated with cooking spray, heat 1½ teaspoons of the oil over medium heat. Drop half of the potato mixture by ¼ cupfuls into the skillet. Flatten into 3" rounds. Cook, turning once, for 6 to 8 minutes, or until golden brown. Transfer to a plate and cover to keep warm.

3. Repeat with the remaining 1½ teaspoons of oil and potato mixture to make 6 pancakes total. Serve the pancakes with the applesauce. Drizzle each serving with the maple syrup.

Per serving: 207 calories, 5 g protein, 32 g carbohydrates, 7 g total fat, 1 g saturated fat, 4 g fiber, 99 mg sodium

Noodle Bowls

Makes 4 servings

¼ cup almond butter

2 tablespoons honey

2 teaspoons reduced-sodium soy sauce

2 teaspoons rice vinegar

2 tablespoons water

2 packages (7 ounces each) shirataki noodles, drained

2 cups shredded cooked chicken breast

¾ cup grated carrots

½ yellow bell pepper, very thinly sliced (about ⅔ cup)

¼ cup sliced almonds, toasted

2–3 radishes, very thinly sliced (about ⅓ cup)

8 scallions, white and some green, thinly sliced (about ½ cup)

2 tablespoons chopped cilantro

1. In a small bowl, combine the almond butter, honey, soy sauce, vinegar, and water.

2. Prepare the noodles according to package directions. Drain, rinse with cold water, and drain thoroughly.

3. In a large bowl, combine the noodles and almond butter mixture, stirring well to coat. Stir in the chicken, carrots, pepper, almonds, radishes, scallions, and cilantro. Divide among 4 bowls and serve.

Per serving: 332 calories, 29 g protein, 23 g carbohydrates, 15 g total fat, 2 g saturated fat, 7 g fiber, 182 mg sodium

Salmon Avocado Wraps

Makes 2 servings

1 can (6 ounces) wild-caught
Alaskan salmon

½ cup chopped scallions

2 tablespoons chopped
fresh parsley

1 tablespoon extra virgin
olive oil

Juice of ½ lime

¼ cup chopped avocado

½ cup cherry tomatoes,
halved

Salt and pepper to taste

4 large bok choy or Chinese
cabbage leaves

In a large mixing bowl, combine the salmon, scallions, parsley, oil, lime juice, avocado, tomatoes, salt, and pepper. Divide the mixture among the bok choy or Chinese cabbage leaves and fold into a wrap. Place 2 wraps on each of 2 plates and serve.

Per serving: 242 calories, 19 g protein, 7 g carbohydrates, 16 g total fat, 3 g saturated fat, 3 g fiber, 326 mg sodium

Hearty Vegetable Soup

Makes 6 servings

1 tablespoon coconut oil

1 pound organic, grass-fed, lean ground beef or shredded cooked chicken

1 onion, chopped

2 cloves garlic, chopped

8 ounces mushrooms, chopped

2 carrots, sliced

2 zucchini, sliced

2 quarts organic chicken or vegetable broth

1 can (14.5 ounces) organic crushed tomatoes

1 can (28 ounces) organic diced tomatoes

1 tablespoon fresh lemon juice (optional)

2 teaspoons dried basil

⅛ teaspoon red-pepper flakes, or to taste

2 cups chopped kale leaves

¼ cup cilantro, chopped

¼ cup fresh parsley, chopped

1. In a stockpot over medium-high heat, heat the oil. Cook the beef or chicken, stirring frequently, for 5 minutes, or until cooked or heated through. Drain and transfer to a plate.

2. In the same pot, cook the onion, garlic, and mushrooms for 5 minutes, or until soft.

3. Stir in the carrots, zucchini, broth, crushed and diced tomatoes, lemon juice (if using), basil, red-pepper flakes, and kale. Cover and simmer for 20 minutes.

4. Add the cilantro and parsley and cover. Simmer for 20 minutes.

Per serving: 287 calories, 23 g protein, 21 g carbohydrates, 13 g total fat, 6 g saturated fat, 5 g fiber, 640 mg sodium

Roasted Chicken and Spinach Salad

Makes 2 servings

2 tablespoons red wine vinegar

2 teaspoons extra virgin olive oil

1 teaspoon Dijon mustard

¼ teaspoon salt

⅛ teaspoon ground black pepper

1 bag (6 ounces) baby spinach

1 boneless, skinless organic chicken breast (about 6 ounces), roasted or grilled and thinly sliced

2 red-skinned pears, cored and thinly sliced

½ red onion, thinly sliced

¼ cup pecans, toasted

1. In a large serving bowl, whisk together the vinegar, oil, mustard, salt, and pepper.

2. Add the spinach, chicken, pears, and onion. Toss to coat well.

3. Divide among 2 plates and top each serving with the pecans.

Per serving: 419 calories, 30 g protein, 41 g carbohydrates, 17 g total fat, 2 g saturated fat, 11 g fiber, 553 mg sodium

Chicken Noodle Soup with Spinach and Basil

Makes 4 servings

1 package (7 ounces) shirataki spaghetti noodles, rinsed and drained

2 tablespoons olive oil

1½ pounds boneless, skinless chicken breasts, cut into bite-size pieces

2 scallions, thinly sliced

1 carton (32 ounces) reduced-sodium organic chicken broth

4 cups spinach leaves, shredded

1 cup basil leaves, shredded

1 tablespoon fresh lemon juice

1. Prepare the noodles according to package directions. Drain and set aside.

2. Meanwhile, in a large saucepan over medium-high heat, heat the oil. Cook the chicken and scallions for 5 minutes, or until lightly browned. Add the broth, reduce the heat to medium, and bring to a simmer. Add the spinach, basil, and lemon juice. Simmer for 4 minutes, or until the spinach is wilted and the chicken is cooked through.

3. Add the reserved noodles to the soup and stir.

Per serving: 288 calories, 29 g protein, 6 g carbohydrates, 11 g total fat, 2 g saturated fat, 2 g fiber, 307 mg sodium

Warm Sweet Potato and Onion Salad with Toasted Walnuts

Makes 4 servings

2 large sweet potatoes (about 2 pounds), peeled and cut into 1" pieces

2 large red onions, cut into wedges

½ teaspoon dried rosemary

½ teaspoon dried oregano

¼ teaspoon salt

¼ teaspoon ground black pepper

1 tablespoon balsamic vinegar

1 teaspoon honey

½ teaspoon Dijon mustard

2 tablespoons sunflower oil

5 cups baby arugula (5 ounces)

20 walnut halves, toasted

1. Preheat the oven to 400°F. Coat a baking sheet with cooking spray.

2. Place the potatoes and onions on the baking sheet and toss with the rosemary, oregano, salt, and pepper. Roast for 30 minutes, turning once, or until tender and browned.

3. In a large bowl, whisk together the vinegar, honey, and mustard. Whisk in the oil. Add the arugula and toss to coat. Toss in the potatoes and onions.

4. Divide the salad among 4 plates and top each serving with the walnuts.

Per serving: 361 calories, 12 g protein, 33 g carbohydrates, 22 g total fat, 7 g saturated fat, 6 g fiber, 377 mg sodium

Fish and Chips

Makes 4 servings

2 sweet potatoes, peeled and cut lengthwise into wedges

1½ teaspoons olive oil

½ teaspoon smoked paprika

⅛ teaspoon salt

¼ teaspoon ground black pepper, divided

1 egg, lightly beaten

1 teaspoon Dijon mustard

⅛ teaspoon ground red pepper

1 cup finely ground almonds or pecans

½ teaspoon dried thyme

4 skinless halibut fillets (6 ounces each)

Lemon wedges or malt vinegar, for serving (optional)

1. Preheat the oven to 425°F. Line 2 large baking sheets with parchment paper.

2. In a large bowl, combine the sweet potatoes, oil, paprika, salt, and ⅛ teaspoon of the black pepper, tossing well to coat. Arrange on 1 of the baking sheets in a single layer. Bake for 15 minutes.

3. Meanwhile, in a shallow dish, whisk the egg, mustard, red pepper, and the remaining ⅛ teaspoon black pepper. In another shallow dish, combine the nuts and thyme. Working with 1 fillet at a time, dip the halibut in the egg mixture, shake off the excess, and then roll in the nut mixture to coat. Place on the second baking sheet. Repeat with the remaining fillets.

4. Remove the potatoes from the oven and toss. Return to the oven with the halibut fillets. Bake for 12 to 15 minutes, or until the halibut is golden and flakes easily.

5. Divide the fish and sweet potatoes among 4 plates. Serve with the lemon wedges or malt vinegar, if using.

Per serving: 278 calories, 35 g protein, 20 g carbohydrates, 6 g total fat, 1 g saturated fat, 2 g fiber, 312 mg sodium

Tangy Roast Beef Lettuce Wraps

Makes 4 servings

¼ cup vegan sour cream

2 teaspoons prepared horseradish, drained

4 large leaves green leafy lettuce

6 ounces thinly sliced roast beef or grilled flank steak

1 apple, cut into 16 slices

1. In a small bowl, combine the sour cream and horseradish until blended.

2. Place the lettuce leaves on a work surface. Spread each leaf with the sour cream mixture. Evenly layer the beef and apple slices down the center of each lettuce leaf. Fold each leaf around the filling and serve.

Per serving: 106 calories, 12 g protein, 8 g carbohydrates, 4 g total fat, 1 g saturated fat, 1 g fiber, 88 mg sodium

Pan-Seared Fish Tacos

Makes 4 servings

1 **Hass avocado, halved, pitted, peeled, and cubed**

3 **tablespoons finely chopped red onion**

2 **tablespoons chopped cilantro**

½ **jalapeño chile pepper, finely chopped (wear plastic gloves when handling)**

1 **tablespoon lime juice**

½ **teaspoon salt, divided**

1 **pound cod fillet, cut into 1" pieces**

1 **teaspoon ground cumin**

½ **teaspoon chili powder**

1 **tablespoon olive oil**

8 **gluten-free tortillas (6" diameter) or lettuce wraps**

1 **cup shredded romaine lettuce**

1. In a small bowl, combine the avocado, onion, cilantro, pepper, lime juice, and ¼ teaspoon of the salt until blended. Set aside. In a medium bowl, toss the cod with the cumin, chili powder, and the remaining ¼ teaspoon salt.

2. In a large nonstick skillet over medium-high heat, heat the oil. Cook the cod for 8 minutes, turning occasionally, or until opaque in the center. Transfer to a plate and keep warm.

3. Wipe out the skillet. Heat the tortillas in the skillet for 30 seconds per side, or according to package directions, until hot and lightly toasted. Dividing evenly, top each tortilla with the romaine, reserved avocado mixture, and cod. Place 2 tacos on each of 4 plates and serve hot.

Per serving: 370 calories, 23 g protein, 39 g carbohydrates, 15 g total fat, 1 g saturated fat, 13 g fiber, 737 mg sodium

Sweet Potatoes Stuffed with Picadillo

Makes 4 servings

4 orange-fleshed sweet potatoes (yams), 6 ounces each

½ pound organic, grass-fed, extra-lean ground beef

1 medium onion, chopped

2 cloves garlic, minced

½ teaspoon dried oregano

¼ teaspoon ground cinnamon

1 can (14.5 ounces) no-salt-added petite diced tomatoes

⅓ cup packed golden raisins (optional)

2 tablespoons no-salt-added tomato paste

¼ teaspoon salt

⅛ teaspoon ground black pepper

1. Preheat the oven to 425°F.

2. Place the sweet potatoes on a baking sheet and roast for 35 minutes, or until easily pierced with a knife.

3. Meanwhile, heat a medium nonstick skillet over medium-high heat. Add the beef, onion, garlic, oregano, and cinnamon. Cook, breaking the beef into smaller pieces with a wooden spoon, for 4 minutes, or until no longer pink. Stir in the diced tomatoes, raisins (if using), and tomato paste. Cook, stirring occasionally, for 5 to 6 minutes, or until slightly thickened. Stir in the salt and pepper.

4. Cut the sweet potatoes in half lengthwise and set 2 halves on each of 4 plates. Top each potato half with ¼ cup of the beef mixture.

Per serving: 307 calories, 16 g protein, 45 g carbohydrates, 8 g total fat, 3 g saturated fat, 7 g fiber, 263 mg sodium

Moroccan Quinoa

Makes 6 servings

1 **cup quinoa**

1 **tablespoon coconut oil**

1 **small onion, finely chopped**

1 **clove garlic, minced**

½ **teaspoon ground coriander**

½ **teaspoon ground cinnamon**

¼ **teaspoon ground turmeric**

Pinch of saffron threads (optional)

1 **cup reduced-sodium vegetable broth**

⅔ **cup water**

1 **tomato, chopped**

⅓ **cup golden raisins**

½ **teaspoon salt**

3 **tablespoons finely chopped fresh parsley**

1. In a fine sieve, rinse the quinoa under cold water for 1 minute. Drain well and set aside.

2. In a large saucepan over medium heat, heat the oil. Cook the onion and garlic, stirring, until softened. Add the coriander, cinnamon, turmeric, and saffron (if using). Cook, stirring constantly, for 30 seconds.

3. Add the reserved quinoa and stir for 1 minute, or until the quinoa is coated with the spices.

4. Add the broth, water, tomato, raisins, and salt and stir to combine. Simmer, covered, for 15 minutes, or until the liquid is absorbed.

5. Remove the saucepan from the heat. Let the mixture stand, covered, for 5 minutes. Stir in the parsley and serve.

Per serving: 167 calories, 5 g protein, 28 g carbohydrates, 4 g total fat, 2 g saturated fat, 3 g fiber, 224 mg sodium

Veggie "Soufflé"

Makes 6 servings

4 cups cauliflower florets (about 1 pound)

6 cups broccoli florets (about 1 pound)

2 teaspoons olive oil

½ cup chopped onion

1 large shallot, finely chopped

1½ cups sliced mushrooms

2 large eggs, divided

4 egg whites, divided

⅔ cup ground pecans, divided

1 teaspoon salt, divided

1 teaspoon ground black pepper, divided

Ground red pepper

1. Preheat the oven to 350°F. Coat an 8" x 4" loaf pan with cooking spray, or use a nonstick loaf pan.

2. In a microwaveable bowl, place the cauliflower and 2 tablespoons of water. Microwave on high power for 6 to 8 minutes, or until soft. Drain off any liquid and set aside.

3. In another microwaveable bowl, place the broccoli and 2 tablespoons of water. Microwave on high power for 3 to 5 minutes, or until soft. Drain off any liquid and set aside.

4. In a large nonstick skillet over medium heat, heat the oil. Cook the onion, shallot, and mushrooms, stirring frequently, for 5 minutes, or until soft. Set aside.

5. In a food processor, combine the reserved cauliflower, 1 egg, 2 egg whites, ⅓ cup of the pecan crumbs, ½ teaspoon of the salt, and ½ teaspoon of the black pepper. Pulse until almost smooth. Scrape into the loaf pan.

6. In the food processor (no need to rinse the bowl after the cauliflower), combine the reserved broccoli and the remaining 1 egg, 2 egg whites, ⅓ cup pecans, ½ teaspoon salt, ½ teaspoon black pepper, and a pinch of red pepper. Pulse until almost smooth.

7. Arrange the reserved mushroom mixture over the cauliflower layer. Gently spread the broccoli mixture over the top. Sprinkle with a pinch of red pepper.

8. Bake for 45 to 50 minutes, or until a wooden pick inserted into the center comes out clean.

Per serving: 193 calories, 10 g protein, 12 g carbohydrates, 13 g total fat, 2 g saturated fat, 6 g fiber, 493 mg sodium

Shepherd's Pie

Makes 4 servings

1¼ pounds sweet potatoes, peeled and cut into 1" pieces

½ cup almond milk

1½ tablespoons coconut oil, divided

¾ teaspoon salt, divided

¼ teaspoon ground black pepper, divided

1 pound organic, grass-fed, lean ground beef

1 medium leek, white part only, washed and chopped (about ½ cup)

1 onion, chopped

2 cups chopped carrots

½ teaspoon dried oregano

½ cup reduced-sodium, fat-free beef broth

¼ cup red wine

¼ cup tomato paste

Ground paprika

1. Preheat the oven to 350°F.

2. Coat a 1½-quart baking dish with cooking spray and set aside.

3. Place the sweet potatoes in a medium pot with enough water to cover by 3". Bring to a boil over medium heat. Lower to a simmer and cook for 10 to 12 minutes, or until tender. Drain the potatoes, return to the pot, and add the almond milk, 1 tablespoon of the oil, ¼ teaspoon of the salt, and ⅛ teaspoon of the pepper. Mash until smooth. Set aside.

4. In a nonstick skillet over medium-high heat, heat the remaining ½ tablespoon oil. Cook the beef, stirring occasionally, for 5 to 6 minutes, or until browned. Drain the fat from the pan and transfer the beef to a bowl.

5. Return the skillet to the heat and add the leek, onion, carrots, and oregano. Cook, stirring occasionally, for 5 to 7 minutes, or until the vegetables are soft.

6. Return the beef to the skillet and stir in the broth, wine, and tomato paste. Cook for 2 to 3 minutes, or until the liquid is almost evaporated. Stir in the remaining ½ teaspoon salt and ⅛ teaspoon pepper.

7. Transfer the beef mixture to the baking dish. Spread the reserved mashed sweet potatoes evenly over the top of the beef. Sprinkle with paprika. Bake for 25 to 30 minutes, or until the potatoes are lightly browned.

Per serving: 363 calories, 29 g protein, 37 g carbohydrates, 10 g total fat, 6 g saturated fat, 7 g fiber, 782 mg sodium

Coconut Vegetable Curry

Makes 4 servings

2 tablespoons extra virgin olive oil

1 tablespoon chopped fresh ginger

1½ teaspoons cumin seeds

3 cups peeled and cubed butternut squash

3 carrots, chopped

½ teaspoon ground turmeric

2 teaspoons ground coriander

1 teaspoon curry powder

1 tablespoon tomato paste

1 can (13.66 ounces) coconut milk

¼ cup water

2 cups frozen peas

1 teaspoon salt

½ cup chopped cilantro

1. In a large pot over medium heat, heat the oil. Cook the ginger and cumin seeds for 1 to 2 minutes, or until the seeds begin to "pop."

2. Add the squash, carrots, turmeric, coriander, and curry powder. Stir well and cook for 1 minute. Add the tomato paste, coconut milk, and water. Stir well.

3. Simmer, covered, for 5 to 10 minutes, or until the squash and carrots are almost done but still a little firm. Add the peas and salt, cover the pot, and simmer for 6 to 7 minutes, or until the vegetables are tender. Remove from the heat and stir in the cilantro.

Per serving: 356 calories, 6 g protein, 26 g carbohydrates, 28 g total fat, 19 g saturated fat, 7 g fiber, 672 mg sodium

Tuscan Tuna Cakes

Makes 4 servings

1 pound yellowfin tuna, cut into ¼" cubes

1 large egg

1 large egg white

¼ cup finely chopped fennel (about ¼ of a medium bulb)

1 small onion, finely chopped

1 tablespoon drained capers

1 tablespoon lemon juice

2 teaspoons grated lemon peel

1 teaspoon chopped fresh oregano

1 cup pine nuts, finely ground

½ teaspoon salt

¼ teaspoon ground black pepper

2 tablespoons olive oil, divided

4 lemon wedges

1. In a large bowl, combine the tuna, egg, egg white, fennel, onion, capers, lemon juice, lemon peel, and oregano. Mix well. Gently fold in the pine nuts, salt, and pepper until just combined.

2. Divide the tuna mixture into 8 equal portions. Shape each into a disk approximately 3½" in diameter and about ½" thick.

3. In a large nonstick skillet over medium heat, heat 1 tablespoon of the oil. Cook 4 tuna cakes for 3 to 4 minutes per side, or until the cakes are golden and cooked through. Repeat with the remaining 1 tablespoon oil and tuna cakes. Serve with the lemon wedges.

Per serving: 448 calories, 34 g protein, 9 g carbohydrates, 32 g total fat, 3 g saturated fat, 2 g fiber, 432 mg sodium

Hearty Winter Harvest Stew

Makes 4 servings

2 tablespoons olive oil

4 boneless, skinless chicken breast halves (about 6 ounces each), cut into ½" pieces

1 onion, chopped

½ cup sliced leek

3 cloves garlic, minced

10 cups peeled and cubed harvest vegetables, such as sweet potatoes, butternut squash, or parsnips

8 cups reduced-sodium chicken broth

2 tablespoons finely chopped fresh ginger

1 tablespoon ground cumin

2 teaspoons sweet paprika

1 teaspoon ground black pepper

½ teaspoon salt

½ teaspoon ground cardamom

3 strips orange peel, white pith removed

2 bay leaves

3 cups winter greens, such as spinach or kale (stems removed), chopped

½ cup snipped fresh Italian parsley

½ cup chopped pistachios, toasted

1. In a large pot over medium-high heat, heat the oil. Cook the chicken, onion, leek, and garlic until lightly browned. Stir in the vegetables, broth, ginger, cumin, paprika, pepper, salt, cardamom, orange peel, and bay leaves. Bring to a boil.

2. Reduce the heat and simmer, uncovered, for 45 to 50 minutes, or until the vegetables are tender. Remove from the heat and discard the bay leaves. Stir in the greens and let wilt. Just before serving, stir in the parsley and pistachios.

Per serving: 254 calories, 23 g protein, 19 g carbohydrates, 9 g total fat, 1 g saturated fat, 4 g fiber, 365 mg sodium

Mock Mashed Potatoes

Makes 4 servings

2 pounds rutabagas, peeled and cubed (approximately 5–6 cups)

2 tablespoons coconut oil

½ cup coconut milk

⅛ teaspoon salt

⅛ teaspoon ground black pepper

1. In a large saucepan over medium-high heat, cook the rutabagas in boiling water for 10 minutes, or until fork-tender. Drain.

2. In a small saucepan over medium-low heat, combine the oil and coconut milk and bring to a slow simmer.

3. Using an electric mixer or food processor, puree the rutabagas until smooth. Add the warmed milk mixture. Blend for 30 seconds, or until creamy. Season with the salt and pepper.

Per serving: 356 calories, 3 g protein, 16 g carbohydrates, 13 g total fat, 11 g saturated fat, 4 g fiber, 97 mg sodium

Grilled Salmon with Citrus Salsa

Makes 4 servings

Salsa

- 2 tablespoons sherry vinegar
- 3 tablespoons extra virgin olive oil
- 1 navel orange, peeled and cut into ¼" pieces
- ½ cup pitted and chopped kalamata olives
- ⅓ cup finely chopped red onion
- ⅓ cup chopped fennel
- 1 tablespoon chopped fresh oregano
- 1 tablespoon chopped Italian parsley

Salmon

- 4 wild-caught salmon fillets (6 ounces each)
- 2 teaspoons extra virgin olive oil

1. *To make the salsa:* In a large bowl, whisk together the vinegar and oil. Stir in the orange, olives, onion, and fennel. Let sit at room temperature while preparing the salmon.

2. *To make the salmon:* Heat a ridged grill pan over medium-high heat. Brush both sides of the salmon lightly with the oil. Grill the salmon, shaking the pan occasionally to keep the fish from sticking and turning once, for 6 to 8 minutes, or until opaque.

3. Transfer the salmon to a serving platter. Add the oregano and parsley to the reserved salsa and spoon evenly over the salmon.

Per serving: 499 calories, 35 g protein, 12 g carbohydrates, 34 g total fat, 5 g saturated fat, 2 g fiber, 135 mg sodium

Pistachio-Crusted Chicken Breasts

Makes 4 servings

2 tablespoons ground
flaxseeds

¾ cup pistachios, crushed to
very fine crumbs

1 tablespoon sliced
almonds, crushed

1 teaspoon dried basil

1 teaspoon dried oregano

1 teaspoon smoked paprika

2 eggs, beaten

4 boneless, skinless chicken
breasts (5–6 ounces each)

1 tablespoon sunflower oil

1. On a large flat plate, combine the flaxseeds, pistachios, almonds, basil, oregano, and paprika and mix well. Pour the eggs in a shallow dish. Dip each chicken breast in the egg and then press both sides of the chicken breasts into the crumb mixture. Make sure the chicken breasts are completely covered in the crumbs.

2. In a 10" skillet over medium heat, heat the oil. Cook the chicken for 8 to 12 minutes, turning once, or until golden brown, a thermometer inserted in the thickest portion registers 165°F, and the juices run clear.

Per serving: 387 calories, 39 g protein, 8 g carbohydrates, 22 g total fat, 3 g saturated fat, 3 g fiber, 208 mg sodium

Beef and Cabbage Stir-Fry

Makes 4 servings

2 tablespoons reduced-sodium soy sauce

2 cloves garlic, minced

1 tablespoon honey

2 teaspoons toasted sesame oil

1 teaspoon hot-pepper sauce

1 teaspoon arrowroot

1 pound organic, grass-fed top sirloin or round steak, sliced across the grain into thin strips

¼ cup unsweetened apple juice

½ cup reduced-sodium beef broth

1 cup chopped onions

3 cups shredded Napa cabbage

1 cup sliced carrots

1. In a shallow glass dish, combine the soy sauce, garlic, honey, oil, hot-pepper sauce, and arrowroot. Add the beef strips and stir. Cover and refrigerate for 30 minutes, stirring occasionally.

2. Heat a large nonstick skillet coated with cooking spray over medium-high heat until hot. Add the beef, reserving the marinade. Cook, stirring, for 5 minutes, or until browned and just slightly pink in the center. Transfer to a plate and cover to keep warm.

3. Add the apple juice and broth to the skillet. Bring to a brisk simmer, scraping the bottom to loosen any browned bits. Add the onions. Cook, stirring, for 1 to 2 minutes, or until the onions are tender. Add the cabbage and carrots. Cook, stirring, for 3 to 4 minutes, or until the vegetables are tender. Return the beef and the reserved marinade to the skillet. Bring to a boil. Cook, stirring, for 1 to 2 minutes, or until the sauce thickens slightly.

Per serving: 237 calories, 27 g protein, 14 g carbohydrates, 8 g total fat, 2 g saturated fat, 2 g fiber, 402 mg sodium

Spaghetti Squash with Stir-Fry Vegetables

Makes 4 servings

1 spaghetti squash (about
  2½–3 pounds)

3 tablespoons sunflower oil

2 cups sliced red bell
  peppers

2 cups broccoli florets

¼ cup Asian garlic chili
  paste

¼ teaspoon red-pepper
  flakes

1 teaspoon toasted
  sesame oil

1. Pierce the skin of the spaghetti squash all over with a small paring knife or fork. Place in a microwaveable dish and microwave on high power for 14 to 20 minutes, turning once, or until the squash is tender and easily pierced. Let stand for 10 minutes.

2. Cut the squash in half lengthwise and remove the seeds. Using a fork, scrape the squash strands into a large serving bowl. Set aside.

3. In a large nonstick skillet over medium-high heat, heat the sunflower oil. Cook the bell pepper and broccoli, tossing frequently, for 5 to 7 minutes, or until the vegetables are tender-crisp. Add the chili paste and red-pepper flakes and stir to coat the vegetables. Cook for 5 minutes. Add the vegetables to the spaghetti squash, toss, and drizzle with the sesame oil.

Per serving: 241 calories, 5 g protein, 23 g carbohydrates, 16 g total fat, 1 g saturated fat, 5 g fiber, 177 mg sodium

Homestyle Roast Beef

Makes 4 servings

2–2½ pounds organic, grass-fed, boneless beef tri-tip roast (bottom sirloin)

1 cup cipollini onions, peeled and sliced

2 cups sliced carrots

2 cloves garlic, minced

1 tablespoon sunflower or olive oil

1 teaspoon dried thyme

1 teaspoon dried oregano

½ teaspoon salt

¼ teaspoon ground black pepper

1 cup reduced-sodium beef broth

1. Preheat the oven to 375°F. Coat the inside of a heavy roasting pan with cooking spray.

2. Place the roast, onions, carrots, and garlic in the pan. Drizzle the oil over the meat and vegetables. Sprinkle on the thyme, oregano, salt, and pepper. With clean hands, toss to coat the vegetables and to rub the seasonings all over the beef.

3. Roast for 50 to 60 minutes, or until a thermometer inserted in the center registers 155°F. Transfer the roast and vegetables to a serving platter. Let stand for 10 minutes.

4. Meanwhile, place the roasting pan over medium heat. Add the broth and cook, scraping the bottom of the pan with a spatula to release the browned particles. Boil for a few minutes to reduce.

5. Slice the roast. Serve the beef and vegetables drizzled with the pan juices.

Per serving: 213 calories, 26 g protein, 8 g carbohydrates, 8 g total fat, 2 g saturated fat, 2 g fiber, 237 mg sodium

Pork Chops and Sweet Potatoes

Makes 4 servings

2 large sweet potatoes,
peeled and cut into
8 wedges each

1 large onion, peeled and
cut into 8 wedges

1 tablespoon sunflower oil

2 teaspoons finely chopped
fresh ginger

¼ teaspoon salt

¼ teaspoon ground
cinnamon

¼ teaspoon ground
black pepper

4 thin-cut boneless pork
chops (about 3 ounces
each)

¼ cup reduced-sodium
vegetable broth or water

1. Preheat the oven to 400°F. Coat a large shallow baking pan with cooking spray. Add the potatoes and onion to the pan.

2. In a small bowl, whisk the oil, ginger, salt, cinnamon, and pepper. Drizzle over the vegetables. With clean hands, rub the seasoning mixture evenly into the vegetables.

3. Bake, tossing occasionally, for 20 to 30 minutes, or until the vegetables start to brown. Reduce the heat to 375°F. Add the pork chops to the pan. Roast for 10 to 15 minutes, or until a thermometer inserted in the center of a chop registers 160°F and the juices run clear. Transfer the pork and vegetables to a serving platter.

4. Add the broth or water to the pan juices and stir to combine, scraping up any bits left in the pan. Pour the pan juices over the pork and vegetables.

Per serving: 332 calories, 18 g protein, 23 g carbohydrates, 19 g total fat, 4 g saturated fat, 4 g fiber, 505 mg sodium

Spaghetti Squash Casserole

Makes 6 servings

1 spaghetti squash
(2½–3 pounds), halved
and seeded

1 tablespoon olive oil

1 small onion, chopped

2 cloves garlic, chopped

2 tablespoons chopped fresh
basil or 1 teaspoon dried

1 can (14.5 ounces) no-salt-
added diced tomatoes

¼ cup chopped fresh parsley

¼ teaspoon salt

¼ teaspoon ground
black pepper

¾ cup pine nuts, lightly
toasted and chopped

1. Preheat the oven to 400°F. Coat a 13" x 9" baking dish and a baking sheet with cooking spray.

2. Place the squash, cut sides down, on the baking sheet. Pierce the skin in a few places with a small paring knife or fork. Bake for 30 minutes, or until tender. With a fork, scrape the squash strands into a large bowl.

3. Meanwhile, in a medium skillet over medium heat, heat the oil. Cook the onion, garlic, and basil for 4 minutes, or until the onion is soft. Add the tomatoes and cook for 5 minutes.

4. Add the parsley, salt, pepper, and the tomato mixture to the bowl with the squash. Toss to coat. Place in the baking dish.

5. Bake for 20 minutes, or until hot and bubbly. Sprinkle with the pine nuts.

Per serving: 201 calories, 4 g protein, 17 g carbohydrates, 15 g total fat, 1 g saturated fat, 4 g fiber, 131 mg sodium

Szechuan Chicken

Makes 4 servings

1 teaspoon minced garlic

1 teaspoon grated
fresh ginger

½ teaspoon salt

¼ teaspoon ground
black pepper

½ teaspoon crushed
fennel seeds

Pinch of ground cloves

1 pound chicken tenders,
cut crosswise into
½"-thick slices

¼ cup sunflower oil

12 ounces bok choy,
cut crosswise into
½"-thick slices

¼ cup reduced-sodium
chicken broth

1 tablespoon gluten-free
tamari

Red-pepper flakes

1. In a large bowl, combine the garlic, ginger, salt, pepper, fennel seeds, and cloves. Add the chicken. With your hands or a fork, toss well to coat all of the pieces with the seasoning.

2. Heat a wok or large skillet over high heat until very hot. Add the oil and swirl to coat the pan. Place the chicken pieces in the pan so they are separated. Cook for 2 to 3 minutes, turning once, or until browned on both sides.

3. Reduce the heat to medium-high. Add the bok choy. Cook, tossing, for 2 minutes, or until the leaves begin to wilt. Add the broth and tamari. Bring to a boil, reduce the heat, and simmer for 2 minutes, or until the chicken is no longer pink and the juices run clear.

4. Garnish with the pepper flakes and serve.

Per serving: 272 calories, 26 g protein, 3 g carbohydrates, 17 g total fat, 2 g saturated fat, 1 g fiber, 637 mg sodium

Frothy Hot Chocolate

Makes 1 serving

1 **cup Almond Breeze unsweetened chocolate almond milk**

1 **teaspoon unsweetened cocoa powder**

4–7 **drops chocolate-flavored SweetLeaf Liquid Stevia Sweet Drops**

In a small saucepan over medium heat, whisk the almond milk, cocoa, and stevia to combine. Bring to a slow boil, reduce the heat, and simmer for 2 minutes, whisking constantly until hot and frothy.

Per serving: 52 calories, 2 g protein, 4 g carbohydrates, 4 g total fat, 0 g saturated fat, 1 g fiber, 180 mg sodium

Marinated Summer Berries

Makes 6 servings

2 cups raspberries

2 cups blueberries

2 cups blackberries

1 cup sliced peaches

4 cups sparkling seltzer or white wine

In a medium bowl, combine the raspberries, blueberries, blackberries, and peaches. Pour the seltzer or wine over the fruit and let stand for 1 hour before serving.

Per serving: 80 calories, 2 g protein, 19 g carbohydrates, 1 g total fat, 0 g saturated fat, 7 g fiber, 1 mg sodium

Baked Apple

Makes 1 serving

1 **Granny Smith apple, cored and cut into 6 wedges**

1 **teaspoon coconut oil**

½ **teaspoon ground cinnamon**

1. Preheat the oven to 425°F.

2. Arrange the apple wedges peel side down on a baking sheet. Drizzle with the oil. Sprinkle with the cinnamon.

3. Bake for 10 to 15 minutes, or until the apple wedges are tender and lightly browned.

Per serving: 151 calories, 1 g protein, 20 g carbohydrates, 9 g total fat, 8 g saturated fat, 4 g fiber, 2 mg sodium

Spiced Pecans

Makes 4 servings

1 cup raw pecans

1 tablespoon honey

1 teaspoon extra virgin olive oil

⅛ teaspoon ground cinnamon

⅛ teaspoon ground ginger

⅛ teaspoon salt

¼ teaspoon ground black pepper

1. Preheat the oven to 300°F.

2. In a small bowl, combine the pecans, honey, and oil. Add the cinnamon, ginger, salt, and pepper and toss to coat. Spread on a baking sheet and bake for 15 minutes, stirring once. Cool slightly before serving.

Per serving: 215 calories, 3 g protein, 8 g carbohydrates, 21 g total fat, 2 g saturated fat, 3 g fiber, 73 mg sodium

Snackin' Nuts

Makes 12 servings

2 **teaspoons olive or sesame oil**

4 **cups mixed raw nuts**

1 **teaspoon garlic powder**

½ **teaspoon ground cumin**

¼ **teaspoon ground turmeric**

1. Preheat the oven to 375°F.

2. In a medium bowl, stir together the oil, nuts, garlic powder, cumin, and turmeric. Spread on a rimmed baking sheet and bake for 12 to 15 minutes, or until toasted.

3. Store the nuts in an airtight container. Keeps for 2 weeks.

Per serving: 231 calories, 4 g protein, 5 g carbohydrates, 24 g total fat, 2 g saturated fat, 3 g fiber, 1 mg sodium

Roasted Kale Chips

Makes 4 servings

2 bunches kale (about 2–2½ pounds), hard stems removed, chopped (about 9 cups chopped)

¼ cup coconut or extra virgin olive oil

¼ teaspoon kosher salt

¼ teaspoon ground black pepper

2 tablespoons nutritional yeast flakes

1. Arrange 3 oven racks evenly spaced apart in the oven. Preheat the oven to 375°F.

2. In a large bowl, toss the kale with the oil, salt, and pepper.

3. Arrange on 3 baking pans or roast kale in batches. (It's important to roast kale with lots of space. If kale is too tight on the pan, it will steam rather than roast and will never get crispy.) Roast for 15 minutes, or until crisp. Sprinkle with the yeast flakes.

Per serving: 207 calories, 8 g protein, 15 g carbohydrates, 16 g total fat, 12 g saturated fat, 4 g fiber, 179 mg sodium

Greens and Fruit Smoothies

Makes 2 servings

1 cup water

3½ cups chopped organic spinach

½ cup chopped fresh parsley

1 banana, frozen

1 pear, cored and chopped

½ cup unsweetened frozen blueberries

2 tablespoons ground golden flaxseed

In a blender, combine the water and spinach. Blend on high speed for 30 seconds to 1 minute, or until smooth. Add the parsley, banana, pear, blueberries, and flaxseed and blend on high speed for 1 minute, or until thoroughly blended.

Per serving: 173 calories, 4 g protein, 36 g carbohydrates, 4 g total fat, 0.5 g saturated fat, 8 g fiber, 49 mg sodium

Baked Pumpkin Pudding

Makes 8 servings

1 can (15 ounces) organic pumpkin

1 can (13.66 ounces) unsweetened coconut milk

¼ cup maple syrup

2 eggs, lightly beaten

1 teaspoon ground cinnamon

¼ teaspoon ground nutmeg

¼ teaspoon ground ginger

1 teaspoon vanilla extract

¾ cup unsweetened almond milk

1. Preheat the oven to 350°F. Lightly coat eight 6-ounce custard cups with cooking spray.

2. In a medium bowl, whisk together the pumpkin, coconut milk, maple syrup, eggs, cinnamon, nutmeg, ginger, vanilla, and almond milk.

3. Divide the mixture among the custard cups. Place the cups in a large baking dish. Fill the dish with water 1" up the sides.

4. Bake for 20 minutes, or until the centers are just barely set.

Per serving: 164 calories, 3 g protein, 13 g carbohydrates, 12 g total fat, 10 g saturated fat, 2 g fiber, 45 mg sodium

Chocolate-Almond Smoothies

Makes 2 servings

1½ cups unsweetened
   almond milk

1 tablespoon maple syrup

1 teaspoon ground flaxseed
   or white chia seeds

1 tablespoon almond butter

1½ teaspoons unsweetened
   cocoa powder

Ice cubes (optional)

1. In a blender, combine the almond milk, maple syrup, flaxseed or chia seeds, almond butter, and cocoa. Blend on high speed for 30 seconds. Let stand for 5 minutes.

2. Blend again on high speed for 30 seconds, or until smooth and frothy. Pour into glasses over ice (if using) and serve.

Per serving: 114 calories, 3 g protein, 11 g carbohydrates, 7 g total fat, 1 g saturated fat, 2 g fiber, 154 mg sodium

Strawberry or Peach Coconut Milk Ice Cream

Makes 4 servings

2 cups fresh or frozen strawberries or peach slices

1 can (13.66 ounces) full-fat unsweetened coconut milk

¼ cup maple syrup

In a blender or food processor, combine the fruit, coconut milk, and maple syrup. Blend or process until combined. Enjoy immediately!

Note: The ingredients can be processed in an ice cream maker for 15 to 20 minutes for a creamier version.

Per serving: 241 calories, 2 g protein, 15 g carbohydrates, 21 g total fat, 18 g saturated fat, 3 g fiber, 15 mg sodium

Avocado Salsa

Makes 4 servings

1 ripe avocado, halved, pitted, and peeled

1 tablespoon finely chopped red onion

2 scallions, minced

1 tablespoon finely chopped jalapeño chile pepper (wear plastic gloves when handling)

1 Roma tomato, seeded and chopped

1 tablespoon lime juice

1 tablespoon coarsely chopped fresh cilantro

1 clove garlic, minced

¼ teaspoon ground cumin

Pinch of salt

Pinch of ground black pepper

Carrot and celery sticks, for serving

1. In a large bowl, mash the avocado. Add the onion, scallions, jalapeño pepper, tomato, lime juice, cilantro, and garlic and stir to combine. Stir in the cumin, salt, and black pepper.

2. Serve with the carrot and celery sticks.

Per serving: 66 calories, 1 g protein, 5 g carbohydrates, 5 g total fat, 1 g saturated fat, 3 g fiber, 114 mg sodium

Nut and Seed Clusters

Makes 8 servings

1 tablespoon ground white chia seeds	¼ teaspoon ground cardamom
3 tablespoons water	½ cup pecans, chopped
1 tablespoon honey	½ cup almonds, chopped
1 teaspoon ground cinnamon	½ cup raw pumpkin seeds (pepitas)
1 teaspoon ground ginger	¼ cup sesame seeds

1. Preheat the oven to 350°F. Line a baking sheet with parchment paper.

2. In a small bowl, soak the chia seeds in the water for 5 minutes.

3. In a medium bowl, whisk the chia seed mixture, honey, cinnamon, ginger, and cardamom. Add the pecans, almonds, pumpkin seeds, and sesame seeds and toss to coat well.

4. Spread the mixture onto the parchment paper. Bake for 20 minutes, or until browned.

5. Cool on a rack for 30 minutes, or until cooled. Break into bite-size pieces.

Per serving: 182 calories, 6 g protein, 8 g carbohydrates, 16 g total fat, 2 g saturated fat, 3 g fiber, 3 mg sodium

Crustless Apple Crumb Pie

Makes 6 servings

5 **Granny Smith apples, peeled, cored, and sliced**

2 **tablespoons maple syrup, divided**

1 **tablespoon lemon juice**

1½ **teaspoons ground cinnamon, divided**

1¼ **cups ground pecans**

¼ **teaspoon ground ginger**

3 **tablespoons Spectrum organic all-vegetable shortening, softened**

1. Preheat the oven to 375°F. Lightly oil a 9" pie plate and set aside.

2. In a large bowl, combine the apples, 1 tablespoon of the maple syrup, the lemon juice, and 1 teaspoon of the cinnamon. Mix gently. Transfer to the pie plate and set aside.

3. In a small bowl, combine the pecans, ginger, shortening, the remaining ½ teaspoon cinnamon, and the remaining 1 tablespoon maple syrup. With clean hands, mix to thoroughly combine.

4. Sprinkle the pecan topping over the reserved apple mixture. Bake for 40 to 45 minutes, or until the fruit is cooked and the topping is browned.

VARIATION: Use 5 cups of peeled and sliced peaches instead of apples and replace the pecans with almonds.

Per serving: 314 calories, 3 g protein, 25 g carbohydrates, 25 g total fat, 5 g saturated fat, 5 g fiber, 2 mg sodium

Peach Melba

Makes 8 servings

4 ripe peaches, halved and pitted

2 teaspoons honey

2 tablespoons Spectrum organic all-vegetable shortening, melted

4 teaspoons raspberry fruit spread, no sugar or artificial sweeteners added

8 mint springs, for garnish (optional)

1. Preheat the oven to 450°F.

2. Place the peach halves cut side up in an 11" x 7" glass baking dish.

3. Brush each peach half with the honey and then with the shortening. Bake for 25 to 30 minutes, or until glazed and very tender. Remove from the oven and let cool for a few minutes.

4. To serve, spoon ½ teaspoon of the raspberry spread into each peach half. Place a peach half on each of 8 dessert plates and garnish each with a mint sprig, if using.

Per serving: 74 calories, 1 g protein, 11 g carbohydrates, 4 g total fat, 2 g saturated fat, 1 g fiber, 0 mg sodium

Eggplant Dip

Makes 6 servings

2 **large eggplants (about 2 pounds total), halved lengthwise**

1 **large onion (unpeeled), halved**

3 **tablespoons lemon juice (from 1½ lemons)**

3 **cloves garlic, minced**

1 **tablespoon tahini (sesame paste)**

1–2 **tablespoons water**

¼ **cup olive oil**

1½ **teaspoons salt**

2 **tablespoons chopped fresh parsley**

1. Preheat the oven to 425°F. Line a baking sheet with foil and brush with olive oil.

2. Place the eggplants and onion cut side down on the baking sheet. Bake for 30 minutes, or until soft and caramelized. Let stand until cool enough to handle.

3. In a medium bowl, combine the lemon juice, garlic, and tahini. Stir in 1 table-spoon of the water. Scrape the seeds from the eggplant and discard. Scrape out the remaining flesh, put in a strainer, and press out as much liquid as possible with the back of a spoon. Add to the bowl. Peel and chop the onion. Add to the bowl.

4. Stir in the oil and salt. Add the remaining 1 tablespoon water if needed to reach desired consistency. Sprinkle with the parsley before serving.

Per serving: 139 calories, 2 g protein, 11 g carbohydrates, 11 g total fat, 1 g saturated fat, 4 g fiber, 587 mg sodium

Elana's Pantry Paleo Chocolate Chip Cookies

Makes 24

2 cups blanched and finely ground almond flour (such as Honeyville)

½ teaspoon baking soda

¼ teaspoon fine sea salt

¼ cup Spectrum organic all-vegetable shortening

3 tablespoons raw, organic honey

1 tablespoon vanilla extract

½ cup chocolate chips

24 pecan halves (optional)

1. Preheat the oven to 350°F. Line 2 large baking sheets with parchment paper.

2. In a food processor, combine the almond flour, baking soda, and salt. Pulse to thoroughly combine. Add the shortening, honey, and vanilla and pulse until thoroughly combined. Remove the blade from the food processor and stir in the chocolate chips.

3. Scoop the dough a tablespoon at a time onto the baking sheets, pressing down to flatten, leaving at least 1" between each cookie. Place a pecan half, if desired, on top of each cookie.

4. Bake for 8 to 11 minutes, or until golden. Let cool on the baking sheets for 5 minutes.

5. Transfer the cookies to racks to cool completely.

Per cookie: 98 calories, 3 g protein, 4 g carbohydrates, 8 g total fat, 2 g saturated fat, 1 g fiber, 54 mg sodium

Endnotes

INTRODUCTION

1   Chuengsamarn S, Rattanamongkolgul S, Luechapudiporn R et al. Curcumin extract for prevention of type 2 diabetes. *Diabetes Care* 2012 Nov;35(11):2121–7.

2   ncbi.nlm.nih.gov/pubmed/?term=extra+virgin+olive+oil+heart+attack.

3   Conrozier T, Mathieu P, Bonjean M et al. A complex of three natural anti-inflammatory agents provides relief of osteoarthritis pain. *Alternative Therapies in Health and Medicine* 2014 Winter;20 Suppl 1:32–7.

4   Basu A, Du M, Leyva MJ et al. Blueberries decrease cardiovascular risk factors in obese men and women with metabolic syndrome. *Journal of Nutrition* 2010 Sep;140(9):1582–7.

CHAPTER 1

1   ismp.org/quarterwatch/pdfs/2012Q4.pdf.

2   Ibid.

3   Light. "Risky Drugs: Why the FDA Cannot Be Trusted." Harvard University. The Lab at Edmond J. Safra Center for Ethics. ethics.harvard.edu/blog/risky-drugs-why-fda-cannot-be-trusted.

4   Ibid.

5   Light D, Lexchin J, Darrow J. Institutional corruption of pharmaceuticals and the myth of safe and effective drugs. *Journal of Law, Medicine & Ethics* 2013 June 1;14(3):590–610.

6   Light. "Risky Drugs." ethics.harvard.edu/blog/risky-drugs-why-fda-cannot-be-trusted.

7   Ibid.

8   Dayantis H. Prediabetes Label 'Unhelpful and Unnecessary.' EurekAlert release, 2014 July 14.

9   medscape.com/viewarticle/825957.

10   diabeteshealth.com/read/2012/08/04/7608/study-shows-turmeric-is-helpful-to-adults-with-prediabetes/.

11   fda.gov/forconsumers/consumerupdates/ucm293330.htm.

12   cdc.gov/chronicdisease/overview/.

13   CDC: Prescription Drug Use Continues to Increase: US Prescription Drug Data, 2007–8. NCHS Data Brief, #42, September 2010.

14   Ibid.

15   Ibid.

16   imshealth.com/ims/Global/Content/Insights/IMS%20Institute%20for%20Healthcare%20Informatics/IHII_Medicines_in_U.S_Report_2011.pdf.

17   Multiple Chronic Conditions among Adults 45+: Trends over the Past 10 Years. NCHS Data Brief, #100, July 2012.

18   gallup.com/poll/145025/americans-doctor-advice-without-second-opinion.aspx.

19   cdc.gov/nchs/fastats/drug-use-therapeutic.htm.

20 bloomberg.com/news/print/2014-04-03/drug-quality-in-china-still-poses-risks
-for-u-s-market.html.

21 medscape.com/viewarticle/828446.

22 joslin.org/info/oral_diabetes_medications_summary_chart.html.

23 nhlbi.nih.gov/health/health-topics/topics/hbp/printall-index
.html; heart.org/HEARTORG/Conditions/HighBloodPressure
/UnderstandYourRiskforHighBloodPressure/Understand-Your-Risk-for-High
-Blood-Pressure_UCM_002052_Article.jsp; medscape.com/viewarticle/804146;
medicinenet.com/hydrochlorothiazide/article.htm.

24 medscape.com/viewarticle/804146.

25 digestive.niddk.nih.gov/ddiseases/pubs/gerd/.

26 medscape.com/viewarticle/825053.

27 cdc.gov/mmwr/preview/mmwrhtml/mm4841a1.htm.

28 nidcr.nih.gov/oralhealth/topics/fluoride/thestoryoffluoridation.htm

29 cdc.gov/mmwr/preview/mmwrhtml/mm4841a1.htm.

30 Ibid.

31 fluoridation.com/c-country.htm.

32 cdc.gov/mmwr/preview/mmwrhtml/mm4841a1.htm.

33 fluoridealert.org/researchers/nrc/findings/.

34 fluoridealert.org/content/europe-statements/.

35 nhlbi.nih.gov/health/health-topics/topics/hbc/causes.html#.

36 archinte.jamanetwork.com/article.aspx?articleid=1861769.

37 Ibid.

38 fda.gov/forconsumers/consumerupdates/ucm293330.htm.

39 Ibid.

40 blogs.psychcentral.com/addiction-recovery/2014/08/three-unlikely-groups-hit
-hard-by-the-prescription-drug-epidemic/.

41 cdc.gov/homeandrecreationalsafety/rxbrief/.

42 samhsa.gov/data/2k13/DAWN079/sr079-Zolpidem.htm.

43 Ibid.

44 drugtopics.modernmedicine.com/drug-topics/news/fda-safety-page-allergic
-reactions-associated-food?page=full.

45 nejm.org/doi/full/10.1056/NEJMc0904562.

46 Morris N. The neglect of nutrition in medical school education: A firsthand look.
JAMA Internal Medicine 2014 June;174(6):841–2.

47 Ibid.

48 Adams KM, Kohlmeier M, Zeisel SH. Nutrition education in US medical schools.
Academic Medicine 2010 Sep;85(9):1537–42.

49 Bredesen D. Reversal of cognitive decline: A novel therapeutic program. *Aging.*
Published online September 27, 2014.

50 Becker Robert O. *The Body Electric,* New York: Morrow, 1985.

51 Lee YW, Chen TL, Shih YR, et al. Adjunctive traditional Chinese medicine
therapy improves survival in patients with advanced breast cancer: a population-
based study. *Cancer* 2014 May 1;120(9):1338–44.

52 Lian F, Li G, Chen X et al. Chinese herbal medicine Tianqi reduces progression from impaired glucose tolerance to diabetes: a double-blind, randomized, placebo-controlled, multicenter trial. *Journal of Clinical Endocrinology & Metabolism* 2014 Feb;99(2):648–55.

CHAPTER 2

1 urmc.rochester.edu/Encyclopedia/Content .aspx?ContentTypeID=134&ContentID=123.

2 madsci.org/posts/archives/1999-07/933464627.An.r.html.

3 cancer.org/cancer/cancerbasics/lymph-nodes-and-cancer.

4 urmc.rochester.edu/Encyclopedia/Content .aspx?ContentTypeID=134&ContentID=123.

5 aaaai.org/conditions-and-treatments/conditions-a-to-z-search/immunoglobulin -e-(ige).aspx.

6 jeeves.mmg.uci.edu/immunology/CoreNotes/Chap21.pdf.

7 med.nyu.edu/content?ChunkIID=21662.

8 emedicine.medscape.com/article/136118-overview.

9 chicagotribune.com/lifestyles/health/sns-201405130000--tms--premhnstr--k -c20140514-20140514-story.html#page=1 (From Harvard Health Letter) 5/14/14.

10 fda.gov/Food/IngredientsPackagingLabeling/FoodAdditivesIngredients /ucm091048.htm.

11 aafa.org/display.cfm?id=9&sub=20&cont=285.

12 medicinenet.com/elisa_tests/article.htm.

13 ncbi.nlm.nih.gov/ pubmed/?term=randomized+double+blind+pilot+study + probiotic+chronic+fatigue+syndrome.

14 ncbi.nlm.nih.gov/pubmed/25048990.

CHAPTER 3

1 amazon.com/s/ref=nb_sb_noss?url=search-alias%3Dstripbooks&field -keywords=diet.

2 amazon.com/s/ref=nb_sb_noss?url=search-alias%3Dstripbooks&field -keywords=diet+chronic+disease.

3 Kushner RF. Barriers to providing nutrition counseling by physicians: a survey of primary care practitioners. *Preventive Medicine* 1995 Nov;24(6):546–52.

4 Kolasa KM. Barriers to providing nutrition counseling by physicians: a survey of primary care practitioners. *Nutrition in Clinical Practice* 2010 Oct;25(5):502–9.

5 healthypeople.gov/2010/.

6 Kolasa KM. Barriers to providing nutrition counseling by physicians. 502–9.

7 en.wikipedia.org/wiki/Hippocrates.

8 Brehm BJ, D'Alessio DA. Benefits of high-protein weight loss diets: enough evidence for practice? *Current Opinion in Endocrinology, Diabetes and Obesity* 2008 Oct;15(5):416–21.

9 Bazzano LA, Hu T, Reynolds K et al. Effects of low-carbohydrate and low-fat diets: a randomized trial. *Annals of Internal Medicine* 2014 Sep 2;161(5):309–18.

10 medicalnewstoday.com/articles/270378.php.

11 hsph.harvard.edu/nutritionsource/omega-3/.

12 ift.org/newsroom/news-releases/2014/september/17/9-fats-to-include-in-a
-healthy-diet.aspx.

13 Fairfield KM, Fletcher RH. Vitamins for chronic disease prevention in adults:
scientific review. *JAMA: The Journal of the American Medical Association* 2002
Jun 19;287(23):3116–26.

14 glycemicindex.com.

15 Brown AC. Gluten sensitivity: Problems of an emerging condition separate from
celiac disease. *Expert Review of Gastroenterology & Hepatology* 2012 Feb;6(1):43–55.

16 Perlmutter David. *Grain Brain,* New York: Little Brown, 2013, 68–9.

17 Brown AC. Gluten sensitivity. 43–55.

18 Ibid.

19 Ibid.

20 Perlmutter David. *Grain Brain,* 50–2.

21 Ibid.

22 Hadjivassiliou M. Gluten sensitivity: from gut to brain. *Lancet Neurology*
2010;9:318–30.

23 Perlmutter D, Vojdani A. Association between headache and sensitivities to
gluten and dairy. *Integrative Medicine* 2013 Apr;12(2).

24 Brown AC. Gluten sensitivity. 43–55.

25 Ibid.

26 Ibid.

27 asaecenter.org/Resources/ANowDetail.cfm?ItemNumber=18644.

28 money.cnn.com/2014/02/24/news/companies/got-milk-ad-dropped/.

29 pcrm.org/health/diets/vegdiets/health-concerns-about-dairy-products.

30 Ibid.

31 digestive.niddk.nih.gov/ddiseases/pubs/lactoseintolerance/index.aspx.

32 rodaleinstitute.org.

33 usda.gov/wps/portal/usda/usdahome?contentidonly=true&contentid=organic
-agriculture.html.

34 whfoods.org/genpage.php?tname=dailytip&dbid=122.

35 journals.cambridge.org/action/displayAbstract?fromPage=online&aid=8491649.

36 ncbi.nlm.nih.gov/pubmed/25045594.

37 sehn.org/ppfaqs.html.

38 whfoods.com/genpage.php?tname=nutrient&dbid=84.

39 whfoods.com/genpage.php?tname=foodspice&dbid=141.

40 prevention.com/food/food-remedies/spices-can-alleviate-common-health
-problems.

41 prevention.com/mind-body/natural-remedies/best-healing-herbs-top-10.

42 water.usgs.gov/edu/propertyyou.html.

43 hsph.harvard.edu/nutritionsource/healthy-drinks/.

44 umm.edu/health/medical/altmed/herb/green-tea.

45 nlm.nih.gov/medlineplus/druginfo/natural/960.html.

46 ncbi.nlm.nih.gov/pubmed/19228856.

47 nlm.nih.gov/medlineplus/druginfo/natural/997.html.

48 prevention.com/print/22241.

49 Floegel A, Pischon T, Bergmann MM et al. Coffee consumption and risk of chronic diseases in EPIC study. *American Journal of Clinical Nutrition* 2012 Apr;95(4):901–8.

50 Bidel S, Hu G, Qiao Q et al. Coffee consumption and risk of total and cardiovascular mortality among patients with type 2 diabetes. *Diabetologia* 2006 Nov;49(11):2618–26.

51 ncbi.nlm.nih.gov/pubmed/25219573.

52 Nestle Marion. *What to Eat,* New York: North Point Press, 2007, 425.

53 Suez J, Korem T, Zeevi D et al. Artificial sweeteners induce glucose intolerance by altering the gut microbiota. *Nature* 2014;514(7521):181–6.

54 webmd.com/alzheimers/news/20110817/moderate-alcohol-drinking-may-cut-alzheimers-risk.

55 bu.edu/today/2013/a-drink-a-day-raises-cancer-risk-study-says/.

56 webmd.com/heart-disease/guide/heart-disease-alcohol-your-heart.

CHAPTER 4

1 cdc.gov/chronicdisease/overview/index.htm.

2 Veerman JL, Healy GN, Cobiac LJ et al. Television viewing time and reduced life expectancy: a life table analysis. *British Journal of Sports Medicine* 2012 Oct;46(13):927–30.

3 hopkinsmedicine.org/healthlibrary/conditions/cardiovascular_diseases/risks_of_physical_inactivity_85,P00218/.

4 Kruk J. Physical activity in the prevention of the most frequent chronic diseases. *Asian Pacific Journal of Cancer Prevention* 2007 Jul–Sep;8(3):325–38.

5 Mons U, Hahmann H, Brenner H. A reverse J-shaped association of leisure time physical activity with prognosis in patients with stable coronary heart disease. *Heart* 2014 Jul;100(13):1043–9.

6 Lian XQ, Zhao D, Zhu M et al. The influence of regular walking at different times of day on blood lipids and inflammatory markers in sedentary patients with coronary artery disease. *Preventive Medicine* 2014 Jan;58:64–9.

7 Di Raimondo D, Tuttolomondo A, Buttà C et al. Metabolic and anti-inflammatory effects of a home-based programme of aerobic physical exercise. *International Journal of Clinical Practice* 2013 Dec;67(12):1247–53.

8 health.harvard.edu/newsletters/Harvard_Mens_Health_Watch/2009/August/Walking-Your-steps-to-health.

9 Ibid.

10 Shiraev T, Barclay G. Evidence based exercise: clinical benefits of high intensity interval training. *Australian Family Physician* 2012 Dec;41(12):960–2.

11 prevention.com/health/diabetes/avoid-belly-fat.

12 aafp.org/afp/2002/0201/p419.html.

CHAPTER 5

1 health.harvard.edu/newsletters/Harvard_Mental_Health_Letter/2011/March /understanding-the-stress-response.

2 Ibid.

3 Rabkin J, Struening E. Life events, stress, and illness. *Science* 1976 Dec;194.

4 Cohen S, Janicki-Deverts D, Doyle W et al. Chronic stress, glucocorticoid receptor resistance, inflammation, and disease risk. *Proceedings of the National Academy of Sciences* 2012 April 2;109(16):5995–9.

5 Cohen S, Tyrrell DA, Smith AP. Psychological stress and susceptibility to the common cold. *New England Journal of Medicine* 1991 Aug 29;325(9):606–12.

6 medicalnewstoday.com/articles/249215.php.

7 eft-help.com/intro/EFThistory.htm.

8 Ortner Nick. *The Tapping Solution*, Hay House, 2013, xii.

9 Ibid.

10 eftuniverse.com/trauma-and-abuse/6-successful-sessions-with-a-war-veteran.

11 Ortner Nick. *The Tapping Solution*, 17–19.

12 heartmath.org.

13 Hirsch JK, Sirois FM, Kitner R. Self-compassion, affect, and health-promoting behaviors. *Health Psychology* 2014 Sep 22.

14 thebuddhistcentre.com/text/loving-kindness-meditation.

15 drweil.com/drw/u/ART00521/three-breathing-exercises.html.

16 relaxationresponse.org.

17 Ibid.

ALLERGIES

1 aaaai.org/conditions-and-treatments/library/at-a-glance/allergic-reactions.aspx.

2 aaaai.org/Aaaai/media/MediaLibrary/PDF%20Documents/Libraries/EL -allergies-colds-allergies-sinusitis-patient.pdf.

3 aaaai.org/conditions-and-treatments/library/at-a-glance/allergic-reactions.aspx.

4 nlm.nih.gov/medlineplus/allergy.html.

5 aafa.org/display.cfm?id=9&sub=24&cont=341.

6 medicinenet.com/fexofenadine-oral/page2.htm.

7 Zeldin DC, Salo PM, Arbes SJ Jr et al. Prevalence of allergic sensitization in the United States. *Journal of Allergy and Clinical Immunology* 2014 Aug;134(2): 350–9.

8 nih.gov/news/health/mar2014/niehs-04.htm.

9 Chatzi L, Apostolaki G, Bibakis I et al. Protective effect of fruits, vegetables and the Mediterranean diet on asthma and allergies among children in Crete. *Thorax* 2007 Aug;62(8):677–83.

10 naturopathic.org/content.asp?contentid=36.

11 naturopathic.org/content.asp?contentid=117.

12 umm.edu/health/medical/altmed/condition/allergic-rhinitis.

13 ncbi.nlm.nih.gov/pubmed/?term=butterbur+cetirizine.

14 Schapowal A. Treating intermittent allergic rhinitis. *Phytotherapy Research* 2005 Jun;19(6):530–7.

15 prevention.com/health/health-concerns/butterbur-spring-allergy-relief.

16 umm.edu/health/medical/altmed/condition/allergic-rhinitis.

17 med.nyu.edu/content?ChunkIID=21574.

18 naturopathic.org/content.asp?contentid=117.

19 Shahar E, Hassoun G, Pollack S. Effect of vitamin E supplementation on the regular treatment of seasonal allergic rhinitis. *Annals of Allergy, Asthma and Immunology* 2004 Jun;92(6):654–8.

20 Altshul S, Loecher B, Faelten S et al. *New Choices in Natural Healing for Women,* Emmaus, PA: Rodale, 1997, 184–7.

21 Naidoo P, Pellow J. A randomized, placebo-controlled pilot study of cat saliva 9cH and Histaminum 9cH in cat allergic adults. *Homeopathy* 2013 Apr;102(2):123–9.

22 Gründling C, Schimetta W, Frass M. Real-life effect of classical homeopathy in the treatment of allergies. *Wiener klinische Wochenschrift* 2012 Jan;124(1–2):11–7.

ARTHRITIS

1 arthritis.org/arthritis-facts/disease-center/.

2 arthritis.org/arthritis-facts/disease-center/osteoarthritis.php.

3 Ibid.

4 arthritistoday.org/about-arthritis/types-of-arthritis/osteoarthritis/treatment -plan/snow-conference-2012.php.

5 arthritistoday.org/about-arthritis/types-of-arthritis/osteoarthritis/who-gets-oa -and-why/cause-of-osteoarthritis.php.

6 arthritisresearchuk.org/arthritis-information/conditions/osteoarthritis/which -joints-are-affected/hands.aspx.

7 arthritistoday.org/about-arthritis/types-of-arthritis/osteoarthritis/who-gets-oa -and-why/cause-of-osteoarthritis.php.

8 fda.gov/downloads/Drugs/DrugSafety/ucm088567.pdf.

9 healio.com/orthopedics/arthritis/news/print/orthopedics- today/%7B2481ef40 -e016-4426-a808-437c567f52ca%7D/research-disputes-effectiveness-of -arthroscopic-surgery-for-knee-oa.

10 ncbi.nlm.nih.gov/pubmed/21121274.

11 ncbi.nlm.nih.gov/pubmed/17137104.

12 Winston David, Kuhn Merrily. *Herbal Therapy & Supplements,* Philadelphia: Lippincott, 2000.

13 umm.edu/health/medical/altmed/herb/ginger.

14 Ying X, Chen X, Cheng S et al. Piperine inhibits IL-β induced expression of inflammatory mediators in human osteoarthritis chondrocyte. *International Immunopharmacology* 2013 Oct;17(2):293–9.

15 umm.edu/health/medical/altmed/condition/osteoarthritis.

16 Altshul S. Docs gone wild. *Prevention* 2014 Oct, 106.

17 umm.edu/health/medical/altmed/condition/osteoarthritis.

18 Altshul S. Docs gone wild. 106.

19 Ibid.

20 consumerlab.com/results/print.asp?reviewid=SAMe.

21 Kim J, Lee EY, Koh EM et al. Comparative clinical trial of S-adenosylmethionine versus nabumetone for treatment of knee osteoarthritis. *Clinical Therapeutics* 2009 Dec;31(12):2860–72.

CARDIOVASCULAR DISEASE

1 strokeassociation.org/STROKEORG/LifeAfterStroke/HealthyLivingAfterStroke /UnderstandingRiskyConditions/Atherosclerosis-and-Stroke_UCM_310426 _Article.jsp.

2 heart.org/HEARTORG/Caregiver/Resources/WhatisCardiovascularDisease /What-is-Cardiovascular-Disease_UCM_301852_Article.jsp.

3 cdc.gov/nchs/fastats/leading-causes-of-death.htm.

4 nhlbi.nih.gov/health/health-topics/topics/hbp/#.

5 Younge JO, Gotink RA, Baena CP et al. Mind-body practices for patients with cardiac disease. *European Journal of Preventive Cardiology* 2014 Sep 16.

6 ncbi.nlm.nih.gov/pmc/articles/PMC3733180/.

7 Xiong XJ, Li SJ, Zhang YQ. Massage therapy for essential hypertension: a systematic review. *Journal of Human Hypertension* 2014 Jul 3.

8 sciencedaily.com/releases/2011/01/110114155241.htm.

9 newsroom.heart.org/news/eating-probiotics-regularly-may-improve-your-blood -pressure.

10 blog.heart.org/seeing-doctor-twice-a-year-helps-keep-blood-pressure-under -control/.

11 nlm.nih.gov/medlineplus/ency/article/000155.htm.

12 nhlbi.nih.gov/health/resources/heart/heart-cholesterol-hbc-what-html.htm.

13 hsph.harvard.edu/nutritionsource/fats-full-story/.

14 Abramson JD, Redberg RF. Don't Give More Patients Statins. *New York Times*, Nov 13, 2013.

15 sciencebasedmedicine.org/statins-the-cochrane-review/.

16 Naci H, Ioannidis J. Comparative effectiveness of exercise and drug interventions on mortality outcomes. *British Medical Journal* 2013;347:f5577.

17 medscape.com/viewarticle/836293.

18 Wu L, Piotrowski K, Rau T et al. Walnut-enriched diet reduces fasting non-HDL-cholesterol and apolipoprotein B in healthy Caucasian subjects. *Metabolism* 2014 March;63(3):382–91.

19 hypertension-cholesterol.com/hypertension-cholesterol/hypertension-1-2557 .html.

20 Lian XQ, Zhao D, Zhu M et al. The influence of regular walking at different times of day on blood lipids and inflammatory markers in sedentary patients with coronary artery disease. *Preventive Medicine* 2014 Jan;58:64–9.

21 Altshul S. Docs gone wild. *Prevention* 2014 Oct, 105.

22 ncbi.nlm.nih.gov/pubmed/11708574.

23 nlm.nih.gov/medlineplus/ency/article/003493.htm.

24 nlm.nih.gov/medlineplus/magazine/issues/summer12/articles/summer12pg6-7.html.

25 mayoclinic.org/diseases-conditions/high-blood-cholesterol/in-depth/cholesterol-levels/art-20048245.

26 medscape.com/viewarticle/750937_2.

27 Anderson JW. Diet first, then medication for hypercholesterolemia. *JAMA: The Journal of the American Medical Association* 2003 Jul 23;290(4):531–3.

28 whfoods.com/genpage.php?tname=disease&dbid=4.

29 feinberg.northwestern.edu/news/2014/06/reverse_heart_disease.html.

30 Ibid.

31 prevention.com/health/health-concerns/best-foods-heart-health?s=25.

32 health.harvard.edu/newsweek/Fabulous_Folate.htm.

33 prevention.com/health/health-concerns/prevent-heart-attacks-best-foods-heart-health.

34 whfoods.com/genpage.php?tname=george&dbid=136.

35 eatright.org/Public/content.aspx?id=6442472548.

36 health.harvard.edu/press_releases/blueberries-strawberries-protect-the-heart.

37 prevention.com/health/health-concerns/best-foods-heart-health.

38 prevention.com/food/healthy-eating-tips/american-heart-association-approved-foods-heart-health/best-fruit-avocado.

39 heart.org/HEARTORG/GettingHealthy/NutritionCenter/HealthyEating/TransFats_UCM_301120_Article.jsphttp://www.heart.org/HEARTORG/GettingHealthy/NutritionCenter/HealthyEating/Trans-Fats_UCM_301120_Article.jsp.

40 health.harvard.edu/newsweek/Fabulous_Folate.htm.

41 newsroom.heart.org/news/high-stress-hostility-depression-linked-with-increased-stroke-risk.

42 eurekalert.org/pub_releases/2014-10/esoc-vd101514.php.

43 Altshul S. Docs gone wild. *Prevention* 2014 Oct, 105.

44 Ibid.

45 Altshul S. Docs gone wild. 106.

46 Naci H, Ioannidis J. Comparative effectiveness of exercise and drug interventions on mortality outcomes. *BMJ* 2013;347:f5577.

47 Rognmo Ø, Hetland E, Helgerud J et al. High intensity aerobic interval exercise is superior to moderate intensity exercise for increasing aerobic capacity in patients with coronary artery disease. *European Journal of Cardiovascular Prevention & Rehabilitation* 2004 Jun;11(3):216–22.

CHRONIC FATIGUE SYNDROME AND FIBROMYALGIA

1 cdc.gov/cfs/symptoms/.

2 anapsid.org/cnd/coping/hillenbrand.html.

3 mayoclinic.org/diseases-conditions/chronic-fatigue-syndrome/basics/treatment/con-20022009.

4 medicinenet.com/script/main/art.asp?articlekey=363&pf=2.

5   medicalnewstoday.com/articles/151139.php.

6   fda.gov/downloads/Drugs/DrugSafety/UCM152825.pdf.

7   themedicalroundtable.com/article/fibromyalgia-new-clinical-concepts.

8   fmswaws.org/medications.html.

9   ods.od.nih.gov/pubs/conferences/ada2002/Milner_abstract.html.

10 Wepner F, Scheuer R, Schuetz-Wieser B et al. Effects of vitamin D on patients with fibromyalgia syndrome. *Pain* 2014 Feb;155(2):261–8.

11 Cordero MD, Alcocer-Gómez E, de Miguel M et al. Can coenzyme q10 improve clinical and molecular parameters in fibromyalgia? *Antioxidants & Redox Signaling* 2013 Oct 20;19(12):1356–61.

12 consumerlab.com/reviews/Acetyl-L-Carnitine-Supplements-Review/Acetyl-L-Carnitine/.

13 Rossini M, Di Munno O, Valentini G et al. Double-blind, multicenter trial comparing acetyl l-carnitine with placebo in the treatment of fibromyalgia patients. *Clinical and Experimental Rheumatology* 2007 Mar–Apr;25(2):182–8.

14 Häuser W, Klose P, Langhorst J et al. Efficacy of different types of aerobic exercise in fibromyalgia syndrome. *Arthritis Research & Therapy* 2010;12(3):R79.

15 ncbi.nlm.nih.gov/pubmed/24018611.

DEPRESSION AND ANXIETY

1   nimh.nih.gov/health/publications/anxiety-disorders/index.shtml.

2   nimh.nih.gov/health/topics/depression/index.shtml.

3   psychcentral.com/lib/depression-versus-anxiety/0001295.

4   ncbi.nlm.nih.gov/pmc/articles/PMC3658370/#__ffn_sectitle.

5   Ibid.

6   adaa.org/understanding-anxiety/generalized-anxiety-disorder-gad.

7   Ibid.

8   adaa.org/understanding-anxiety/generalized-anxiety-disorder-gad/symptoms.

9   nimh.nih.gov/health/topics/panic-disorder/index.shtml.

10 acceleratedresolutiontherapy.com.

11 ncbi.nlm.nih.gov/pubmed/24306011.

12 Kip KE et al. RCT accelerated resolution therapy (ART) for PTSD. *Military Medicine* 2013 Dec;178(12):1298–309.

13 adaa.org/finding-help/treatment/medication.

14 Ibid.

15 nlm.nih.gov/medlineplus/druginfo/meds/a694020.html.

16 nlm.nih.gov/medlineplus/druginfo/meds/a604030.html.

17 nlm.nih.gov/medlineplus/druginfo/meds/a694020.html.

18 nlm.nih.gov/medlineplus/druginfo/meds/a604030.html.

19 cdc.gov/mmwr/preview/mmwrhtml/mm6340a1.htm?s_cid=mm6340a1_x.

20 medscape.com/viewarticle/831403.

21 medscape.com/viewarticle/771951.

22 drugs.com/stats/top100/sales.

23 medicinenet.com/aripiprazole/article.htm.

24 nytimes.com/2012/09/25/health/a-call-for-caution-in-the-use-of-antipsychotic
    -drugs.html.

25 Osher Y, Belmaker RH. Omega-3 fatty acids in depression. *CNS Neuroscience
    Therapy* 2009 Summer;15(2):128–33.

26 Somer Elizabeth. *Food & Mood,* New York: Holt, 1999.

27 beckinstitute.org/cognitive-behavioral-therapy/.

28 Ibid.

29 medscape.com/viewarticle/832762?nlid=67184_2863&src=wnl_edit_dail.

30 socialanxietyinstitute.org/dsm-definition-social-anxiety-disorder.

31 medscape.com/viewarticle/832762?nlid=67184_2863&src=wnl_edit_dail.

32 medicalnewstoday.com/articles/232248.php#natural_ways_to_boost
    _serotonin_levels.

33 adaa.org/living-with-anxiety/managing-anxiety/exercise-stress-and-anxiety.

34 Ibid.

35 Ibid.

36 emedexpert.com/compare/ssris-vs-tca.shtml.

37 medicalnewstoday.com/articles/281830.php.

38 Angoa-Pérez M, Kane MJ, Briggs DI et al. Mice genetically depleted of brain
    serotonin do not display a depression-like behavioral phenotype. *ACS Chemical
    Neuroscience* 2014;5(10):908–19.

39 nccaom.org.

40 med.nyu.edu/content?ChunkIID=653856.

41 ncbi.nlm.nih.gov/pubmed/21208586.

42 umm.edu/health/medical/altmed/supplement/vitamin-b1-thiamine.

43 prevention.com/mind-body/natural-remedies/vitamin-b12-and-depression.

44 prevention.com/mind-body/natural-remedies/herbs-and-supplements-natural
    -remedies-doctors-prescribe.

45 prevention.com/same.

46 jad-journal.com/article/S0165-0327(14)00362-0/abstract.

47 consumerlab.com/reviews/turmeric-curcumin-supplements-spice-review
    /turmeric/.

48 Amsterdam JD, Shults J, Soeller I et al. Chamomile (*Matricaria recutita*) may
    provide antidepressant activity in anxious, depressed humans. *Alternative
    Therapies in Health and Medicine* 2012 Sep–Oct;18(5):44–9.

49 vitacost.com/natures-way-chamomile-standardized.

DIABETES

1   cdc.gov/vhf/Ebola/outbreaks/2014-west-africa/index.html.

2   Ibid.

3   nytimes.com/interactive/2014/07/31/world/africa/ebola-virus-outbreak-qa.html.

4   diabetes.org/diabetes-basics/statistics.

5   ucl.ac.uk/news/news-articles/0714/010714-Diabetes-treatments-do-more-harm
    -than-good.

6   Yudkin JS, Montori VM. The epidemic of pre-diabetes: The medicine and the
    politics. *British Medical Journal* 2014;349:g4485.

7   natap.org/2009/HIV/010509_05.htm.

8   Moore EM, Mander AG, Ames D et al. Increased risk of cognitive impairment
    in patients with diabetes is associated with metformin. *Diabetes Care* 2013
    Oct;36(10):2981–7.

9   medicinenet.com/hyperglycemia/article.htm.

10 Outsmart diabetes. *Prevention* 2013 Jun 11, 16.

11 annals.org/article.aspx?articleid=474081.

12 Akbaraly T, Sabia S, Hagger-Johnson G et al. Does overall diet in midlife predict
    future aging phenotypes? *American Journal of Medicine* 2013 May;126(5):411–9.e3.

13 Altshul S. Get a leg up on diabetes. *Prevention* 2013 Mar, 78.

14 diabetes.niddk.nih.gov/dm/pubs/preventionprogram.

15 ymca.net/diabetes-prevention/.

16 cdc.gov/diabetes/prevention/recognition/states/Pennsylvania
    .htm?choice=states%2FPennsylvania.htm.

17 Feinman RD, Pogozelski WK, Astrup A et al. Dietary carbohydrate restriction as
    the first approach in diabetes management: Critical review and evidence base.
    Nutrition 2015 Jan;31(1):1–13.

18 medscape.com/viewarticle/831161.

19 Gulati S, Misra A, Pandey RM et al. Effects of pistachio nuts on body
    composition, metabolic, inflammatory and oxidative stress parameters in Asian
    Indians with metabolic syndrome. *Nutrition* 2014 Feb;30(2):192–7.

20 jn.nutrition.org/content/138/9/1752S.full.

21 Altshul S. Outsmart diabetes. *Prevention* 2013 Jun 11, 29.

22 Altshul S. Docs gone wild. *Prevention* 2014 Oct, 106.

23 Altshul S. Docs gone wild. 108.

24 Witte AV, Kerti L, Margulies DS et al. Effects of resveratrol on memory
    performance, hippocampal functional connectivity, and glucose metabolism in
    healthy older adults. Journal of Neuroscience 2014 Jun 4;34(23):7862–70.

25 Bhatt JK, Thomas S, Nanjan MJ. Resveratrol supplementation improves glycemic
    control in type 2 diabetes mellitus. *Nutrition Research* 2012 Jul;32(7):537–41.

26 Altshul S. Outsmart diabetes. *Prevention* 2013 Mar 12, 40–1.

ECZEMA AND PSORIASIS

1   emedicine.medscape.com/article/1943419-overview.

2   medicalnewstoday.com/articles/14417.php.

3   uchospitals.edu/specialties/dermatology/light-therapy/.

4   ncbi.nlm.nih.gov/pubmed/10767672.

5   med.nyu.edu/content?ChunkIID=104391.

6   ncbi.nlm.nih.gov/pubmed/16148424.

7   ewg.org.

8   Millsop JW, Bhatia BK, Debbaneh M et al. Diet and psoriasis, part III: Role of nutritional supplements. *Journal of the American Academy of Dermatology* 2014 Sep;71(3):561–9.

9   emedicine.medscape.com/article/1943419-overview.

10 medicalnewstoday.com/articles/14417.php.

HEADACHES AND MIGRAINES

1   nccam.nih.gov/sites/nccam.nih.gov/files/D462.pdf.

2   ncbi.nlm.nih.gov/pubmedhealth/PMH0001728/.

3   Ramsden CE, Faurot KR, Zamora D et al. Targeted alteration of dietary n-3 and n-6 fatty acids for the treatment of chronic headaches. *Pain* 2013 Nov;154(11):2441–51.

4   Altshul Sara. *Woman's Book of Healing Herbs,* Emmaus, PA: Rodale, 1999, 241.

5   headaches.org/content/headache-sufferers-diet.

6   Ibid.

7   emedicine.medscape.com/article/1142556-treatment.

8   Shamliyan TA, Choi JY, Ramakrishnan R et al. Preventive pharmacologic treatments for episodic migraine in adults. *Journal of General Internal Medicine* 2013 Sep;28(9):1225–37.

9   emedicine.medscape.com/article/1142556-treatment.

10 Lawler SP, Cameron LD. A randomized, controlled trial of massage therapy as a treatment for migraine. *Annals of Behavioral Medicine* 2006 Aug;32(1):50–9.

11 Arnadottir TS, Sigurdardottir AK. Is craniosacral therapy effective for migraine? *Complementary Therapies in Clinical Practice* 2013 Feb;19(1):11–4.

12 Wells RE, Burch R, Paulsen RH et al. Meditation for migraines: A pilot randomized controlled trial. *Headache* 2014 Oct;54(9):1484–95.

13 Mauskop Alexander. *What Your Doctor May Not Tell You about Migraines,* New York: Warner, 2001.

14 Altshul S. Docs gone wild. *Prevention* 2014 Oct, 106.

15 Pareek A, Suthar M, Rathore GS et al. Feverfew: A systematic review. *Pharmacognosy Reviews* 2011 Jan–Jun;5(9):103–10.

16 http://umm.edu/health/medical/altmed/herb/feverfew.

17 Maghbooli M, Golipour F, Moghimi Esfandabadi A et al. Comparison between the efficacy of ginger and sumatriptan in the ablative treatment of the common migraine. *Phytotherapy Research* 2014 Mar;28(3):412–5.

IBS AND GERD

1   digestive.niddk.nih.gov/ddiseases/pubs/ibs/.

2   Newman Alvin. *The Essential IBS Book,* Toronto: Robert Rose, 2011, 13.

3   http://digestive.niddk.nih.gov/ddiseases/pubs/ibs/.

4   Newman Alvin. *The Essential IBS Book,* 26.

5   emedicine.medscape.com/article/179037-overview.

6   health.clevelandclinic.org/2014/02/take-control-of-ibs-with-low-fodmap-diet/.

7   patient.co.uk/health/irritable-bowel-syndrome-diet-sheet.

8   Fujimura KE, Slusher NA, Cabana MD et al. Role of the gut microbiota in defining human health. *Expert Review of Anti-Infective Therapy* 2010 April;8(4):435–54.

9   academy.asm.org/images/stories/documents/FAQ_Human_Microbiome.pdf.

10 mayoclinicproceedings.org/article/S0025-6196(13)00886-0/pdf.

11 Suarez K, Mayer C, Ehlert C et al. Psychological stress and self-reported functional gastrointestinal disorders. *Journal of Nervous and Mental Disease* 2010 Mar;198(3):226–9.

12 health.harvard.edu/newsletters/Harvard_Mental_Health_Letter/2010 /August/stress-and-the-sensitive-gut?utm_source=mental&utm _medium=pressrelease&utm_campaign=mental0810.

13 ncbi.nlm.nih.gov/pubmed/?term=progressive+muscle+relaxation+IBS.

14 Suarez K. Psychological stress and self-reported functional gastrointestinal disorders. 226–9.

15 health.harvard.edu/newsletters/Harvard_Mental_Health_Letter/2010 /August/stress-and-the-sensitive-gut?utm_source=mental&utm _medium=pressrelease&utm_campaign=mental0810.

16 Altshul S. Docs gone wild. *Prevention,* Oct 2014, 109–10.

17 Vanuytsel T, Tack JF, Boeckxstaens GE. Treatment of abdominal pain in irritable bowel syndrome. *Journal of Gastroenterology* 2014 Aug;49(8):1193–205.

18 drweil.com/drw/u/ART00680/Irritable-Bowel-Syndrome-IBS.html.

19 Kuhn Merrily, Winston David. *Herbal Therapy & Supplements,* Philadelphia: Lippincott, 2000.

20 medscape.com/viewarticle/804146.

21 digestive.niddk.nih.gov/ddiseases/pubs/gerd/.

INSOMNIA

1   Masters P. In the clinic: Insomnia. *Annals of Internal Medicine* 2014;161(7):ITC1.

2   Ibid.

3   Editors of *Prevention. The Belly Melt Diet,* Emmaus, PA: Rodale, 2012, 36–7.

4   prevention.com/health/health-concerns/how-lack-sleep-increases-your-alzheimers-risk.

5   ninds.nih.gov/disorders/brain_basics/understanding_sleep.htm.

6   medicalnewstoday.com/articles/232248.php.

7   functionalmedicineuniversity.com/public/906.cfm.

8   fda.gov/downloads/Drugs/DrugSafety/UCM335007.pdf.

9   Ibid.

10 nlm.nih.gov/medlineplus/druginfo/meds/a693025.html.

11 medscape.com/viewarticle/831403.

12 mirecc.va.gov/visn4/bhl/docs/benzodiazepines.pdf.

13 Lin HH, Tsai PS, Fang SC et al. Effect of kiwifruit consumption on sleep quality in adults with sleep problems. *Asia Pacific Journal of Clinical Nutrition* 2011;20(2):169–74.

14 psychologytoday.com/blog/sleep-newzzz/201311/kiwi-super-food-sleep.

15 Grandner MA, Kripke DF, Naidoo N et al. Relationships among dietary nutrients and subjective sleep, objective sleep, and napping in women. *Sleep Medicine* 2010 Feb;11(2):180.

16 health.clevelandclinic.org/2014/06/5-foods-that-help-you-sleep/.

17 doctormurray.com/health-conditions/insomnia-sleep-wake-cycle-disorder/.

18 sleepfoundation.org/sleep-news/food-could-keep-you-awake.

19 umm.edu/health/medical/altmed/condition/insomnia.

20 Passos GS, Poyares D, Santana MG et al. Exercise improves immune function, antidepressive response, and sleep quality in patients with chronic primary insomnia. *BioMed Research International* 2014, article ID 498961.

21 Khalsa SB. Treatment of chronic insomnia with yoga. *Applied Psychophysiology and Biofeedback* 2004 Dec;29(4):269–78.

22 umm.edu/health/medical/altmed/condition/insomnia.

23 ncbi.nlm.nih.gov/pubmed/23853635.

MENOPAUSE

1 pubs.acs.org/subscribe/archive/mdd/v03/i08/html/kling.html.

2 peta.org/issues/animals-used-for-experimentation/animals-used -experimentation-factsheets/premarin-prescription-cruelty/#ixzz3HN9eDxFg.

3 Herber-Gast GC, Mishra GD. Fruit, Mediterranean-style, and high-fat and -sugar diets are associated with the risk of night sweats and hot flushes in midlife. *American Journal of Clinical Nutrition* 2013 May;97(5):1092–9.

4 whfoods.com/genpage.php?tname=newtip&dbid=36.

5 Ross SM. Menopause: a standardized isopropanolic black cohosh extract (remifemin) is found to be safe and effective for menopausal symptoms. *Holistic Nursing Practices* 2012 Jan–Feb;26(1):58–61.

6 Stojanovska L, Apostolopoulos V, Polman R et al. To exercise, or, not to exercise, during menopause and beyond. *Maturitas* 2014 April;77(4):318–23.

7 prevention.com/health/health-concerns/activity-linked-fewer-night-sweats -menopause.

8 baylor.edu/mediacommunications/news.php?action=story&story=147581.

9 prevention.com/health/health-concerns/natural-remedies-hot-flashes.

10 my.clevelandclinic.org/health/diseases_conditions/hic-what-is-perimenopause -menopause-postmenopause/hic_Menopause_and_Osteoporosis.

11 Chiu HY, Pan CH, Shyu YK et al. Effects of acupuncture on menopause-related symptoms and quality of life in women on natural menopause. *Menopause* 2014 Jul 7.

12 nccaom.org.

OBESITY

1 Ladabaum U, Mannalithara A, Myer PA et al. Obesity, abdominal obesity, physical activity, and caloric intake in US adults: 1988 to 2010. *American Journal of Medicine* 2014 Aug;127(8):717–27.

2 win.niddk.nih.gov/publications/PDFs/stat904z.pdf.

3   Simmons AL, Schlezinger JJ, Corkey BE. What are we putting in our food that is making us fat? *Current Obesity Reports* 2014 Jun 1;3(2):273–85.

4   Ibid.

5   Kemps E, Tiggemann M, Hollitt S. Exposure to television food advertising primes food-related cognitions and triggers motivation to eat. *Psychology & Health* 2014;29(10):1192–205.

6   prevention.com/food/healthy-eating-tips/eating-pepper-helps-you-eat-fewer -calories.

7   prevention.com/print/50096.

8   drweil.com/drw/u/ART00521/three-breathing-exercises.html.

9   prevention.com/mind-body/natural-remedies/safety-herbal-supplements?page =3&cm_BULbczB8WctNB879b%24ADD8jS47h=1412283273&cm _BUPYW3B8WctNB879b%24ADD8jS3oh=1413319480.

10 Public Health England, 2014 Jul 31. Adult obesity and type 2 diabetes.

SINUSITIS

1   nlm.nih.gov/medlineplus/sinusitis.html.

2   pacificcollege.edu/acupuncture-massage-news/articles/1126-improve-your -sinuses-today-what-to-eat-to-avoid-inflammation.html.

3   naturopathconnect.com/articles/sinusitis-dietary/.

4   ncbi.nlm.nih.gov/pubmed/22112724.

5   umm.edu/health/medical/altmed/herb/elderberry.

6   ncbi.nlm.nih.gov/pubmed/25117505.

7   umm.edu/health/medical/altmed/condition/sinusitis.

Index

Underscored page references indicate sidebars and tables. **Boldface** references indicate photographs.

Breathing exercise, for stress reduction, 113, 235–36
Broccoli
Spaghetti Squash with Stir-Fry Vegetables, 285
Veggie "Soufflé," 274–75
Brussels sprouts, for heart health, 146
Butterbur, for treating
allergy symptoms, 125
headaches and migraines, 196, 198
Butternut squash
Coconut Vegetable Curry, 278
Hearty Winter Harvest Stew, 280
B vitamins, for treating anxiety and depression, 169, 173

C

Cabbage
Beef and Cabbage Stir-Fry, 284
Salmon Avocado Wraps, 264
Caffeine avoidance, during stress, 235
Calcium
in dairy products, 55
for osteoporosis prevention, 227
sleep-promoting, 216
Cancer. *See also specific types of cancer*
deaths from, 139
from hormone replacement therapy, 221
inactivity and, 75
from pesticides, 57
preventing, 61, 62, 64–65, 224
Candles, scented, 124
Carbohydrate restriction, in No More Pills Plan, 49
Cardiologist, when to see, 151
Cardiovascular disease. *See also* Heart disease
contributors to, 138–45 (*see also* Cholesterol; High blood pressure)
definition of, 138
No More Pills Plan preventing, 138
Carrots
Coconut Vegetable Curry, 278
Hearty Vegetable Soup, 265
Casein allergy, 36, 37, 55–56
Cataracts, from statin drugs, 143
Cat-Cow (yoga pose), 97, 97
Cauliflower
Veggie "Soufflé," 274–75
CBT. *See* Cognitive behavioral therapy
Celiac disease, 37, 52–53, 54
CFIDS (chronic fatigue immune deficiency syndrome), 152
CFS. *See* Chronic fatigue syndrome

Chair massage, for blood pressure reduction, 140
Chair Squats, 82
Chamomile, for treating
anxiety, 174–75
IBS, 207
Chia seeds
for heart health, 147
Nut and Seed Clusters, 301
Chicken
Chicken Noodle Soup with Spinach and Basil, 267
Hearty Winter Harvest Stew, 280
Pistachio-Crusted Chicken Breasts, 283
Roasted Chicken and Spinach Salad, 266
Szechuan Chicken, 289
Child's Pose, 97, 98, **98**, 101
Chinese herbs, for treating
anxiety and depression, 172
knee pain, 137
Chocolate, 59
Chocolate-Almond Smoothies, 298
Elana's Pantry Paleo Chocolate Chip Cookies, 305
Frothy Hot Chocolate, 290
Cholesterol
excess buildup of, 16, 141
HDL (*see* HDL cholesterol)
high, causes of, 12
LDL, 141, 148
lowering, with
cinnamon, 62
diet, 141–42, 143
green tea, 64
No More Pills Plan, 143–44
red yeast rice, 144
statins, 12, 16–18, 142–43
walking, 76, 143
measurements of, 144
roles of, 141
Chronic conditions, from delayed-type food allergies, 31–32
Chronic diseases. *See also specific diseases*
basics for treating, 6
causes of, 9, 10–11
inactivity, 74
inflammation, 42, 48
modern American lifestyle, 8–9
vitamin D deficiency, 42
exercise decreasing, 75, 76
problems of drugs for, 12–13
statistics on, 10
stress linked to, 102, 105–6
Chronic fatigue immune deficiency syndrome (CFIDS), 152

Chronic fatigue syndrome (CFS). *See also*
    Fibromyalgia
    exercising with, 158–59, <u>158</u>
    possible triggers of, <u>153</u>
    symptoms of, 152, <u>153</u>, 154
    treating, with
        cognitive behavioral therapy, <u>159</u>
        drugs, 154, 155
        No More Pills Plan, 156–57
Cinnamon, health benefits of, 62
Cleaning products, allergies from, 124
Clear Sinus and Ear, for sinusitis, 249
Cobra (yoga pose), 99, **99**
Coconut milk
    Coconut Vegetable Curry, 278
    Strawberry or Peach Coconut Milk Ice
        Cream, 299
Cod
    Pan-Seared Fish Tacos, 271
Coenzyme Q10
    for heart health, 150
    for treating
        chronic fatigue syndrome, 157–58
        fibromyalgia, 157–58
Coffee
    avoiding, during stress, 235
    for diabetes prevention, 183
    health benefits of, 66–67
Cognitive behavioral therapy (CBT), for
        treating
    anxiety and depression, 169–70
    chronic fatigue syndrome, <u>159</u>
    emotional eating, 242
    fibromyalgia, 156, <u>159</u>
    IBS, 206
    panic disorder, 164
    post-traumatic stress disorder, 164
Colds, symptoms of, <u>120</u>
Colon cancer
    gluten sensitivity and, 35
    preventing, 61, 75
Compassion exercise, for stress reduction,
        111–13
Constipation, <u>202</u>
Cookies
    Elana's Pantry Paleo Chocolate Chip
        Cookies, 305
Coronary artery disease, walking preventing,
        76
Corticosteroid inhalers, side effects of, 121
Cortisol levels
    massage reducing, 197
    stress increasing, 105, 235
Craniosacral therapy, for treating headaches
        and migraines, 197
Curcumin. *See also* Turmeric
    for diabetes prevention, xi, 8

for treating
    anxiety and depression, 174
    arthritis, 134, 136
    IBS, 207
    inflammation, 104
Curry powder
    Coconut Vegetable Curry, 278

D

Dairy foods, problems from, 37, 54–56
Dairy-free diet
    No More Pills Plan as, 54–56, 60
    for treating arthritis, <u>133</u>
Deadlift Curl Press, 92–93, **92–93**
Death
    causes of
        diabetes, 176
        diseases, 10, <u>139</u>
        prescription drugs, 3, 4, 10, 18
        smoking, 11
    walking preventing, 76
Depression
    cardiovascular health and, <u>149</u>
    causes of, 162, 165
    fibromyalgia and, <u>160</u>
    inactivity and, 75
    incidence of, 161
    ineffective treatment of, 161–62
    with seasonal affective disorder, <u>175</u>
    serotonin and, <u>170–71</u>
    symptoms of, 161, 162
    treating, with
        cognitive behavioral therapy, 169–70
        medications, 165–68
        No More Pills Plan, 168–69
        physical activity, 170–72
        supplements, 172–75
        traditional Chinese medicine, 172
Desserts. *See* Snacks and desserts
D-Hist, for sinusitis, 249
Diabetes, type 1, 178, 180
Diabetes, type 2. *See also* Prediabetes
    bariatric surgery and, <u>241</u>, <u>242</u>
    belly fat and, 78
    case study about, <u>182</u>
    causes of, <u>12</u>, 17, 50, 68, 176
    controlling, with
        exercise, 184–85
        green tea, 65
        No More Pills Plan, 180–81, 183
        prescription drugs, <u>12–13</u>, 177
        supplements, 183–84
        traditional Chinese medicine, 27–28
    development of, 178
    epidemic of, 176

4-7-8 Breathing Exercise, for stress
reduction, 113, 235–36
FPIES (food protein-induced enterocolitis
syndrome), 201
Freeze-Frame technique, for stress reduction,
110
Fruits. *See also specific fruits*
fiber in, 49
Greens and Fruit Smoothies, 296
for headache prevention, 195
for menopause symptom relief, 225
organic, 58
underconsumption of, 10

G

GAD (generalized anxiety disorder), 163
Garlic, for heart health, 147
Gastroesophageal reflux disease. *See* GERD
Gastrointestinal tract, <u>203</u>, 205–6
GDH (gut-directed hypnotherapy), for
treating digestive problems, 206
Generalized anxiety disorder (GAD), 163
Genes, osteoarthritis-related, 130
Genetically modified (GMO) produce, 57–58
GERD
causes of, <u>13</u>, 201, 208, 209, <u>209</u>, <u>210</u>
symptoms of, 53, 208
treating, <u>13</u>, 210
Ginger
for headache prevention, 195
health benefits of, 61–62
for treating
arthritis, 134–35
headaches and migraines, 199–200
Glucosamine/chondroitin, for treating
arthritis, 136
Gluten
facts about, 52–54
insomnia from, 218–19
Gluten-free diet, No More Pills Plan as, 51–52
Gluten-free foods
as recipe ingredients, 253
in restaurants, <u>211</u>
Gluten intolerance, strokes from, 51
Gluten sensitivity, 35, 37, 53, 54
Glycemic index, 51
GMO produce, 57–58
Grains
avoiding, in No More Pills Plan, 50, 60
gluten in, 52, 54
Grapefruit
Honey-Sweet Broiled Grapefruit Halves,
259

Green tea, health benefits of, 63–65, 66
Guided imagery, for stress reduction,
110–11
Gut-directed hypnotherapy (GDH), for
treating digestive problems, 206

H

Halibut
Fish and Chips, 269
Hand pain, from arthritis, <u>133</u>
Hay fever, 121. *See also* Allergies
HDL cholesterol
diabetes risk and, 179
increasing, 64, 69, 144–45
trans fats lowering, 148
Headaches. *See also* Migraines
common causes of, 193
preventing, 195, 197
tension, 193, <u>200</u>
treatments for, 196–200
triggers of, 53, 194–96
Heart attacks
from Prempro, 221
preventing, xii, 9, 64, 65, 76
vitamin D deficiencies and, 148–49
Heart disease. *See also* Cardiovascular
disease
deaths from, <u>139</u>
effect of exercise on, 75
emotional contributors to, <u>149</u>
family history of, <u>151</u>
inactivity and, 74
preventing, with
coffee, 66–67
diet, 49–50, 145, 146–48
exercise, 150–51
statins, 9
supplements, 148–50
reversing, 145–46
trans fats promoting, 147–48
HeartMath, for stress reduction, 109–10
HEPA filters, 124
Herbal teas, <u>64</u>
Herbs, in No More Pills Plan, 61, 62. *See also*
specific herbs
High blood pressure
alcohol and, 69–70, <u>141</u>
causes of, <u>13</u>, 16, <u>141</u>
as diabetes risk factor, 178
facts about, 138–39
inactivity and, 74
methods of lowering, xii, 64, 139–41
treatment side effects and, <u>13</u>

High blood sugar. *See also* Blood sugar
    levels
    author's experience with, 45–46
    from carbohydrates, 49
    complications from, 178
    from exercise-induced stress, 185
    reducing, with
        interval training, 46, 185, 234
        No More Pills Plan, 181
        supplements, 183–84
        vinegar, 183, 234
    from statins, 17
High cholesterol. *See* Cholesterol
High-fiber diet, No More Pills Plan as,
    49–50
Hillenbrand, Laura, 153
Histamines, allergy symptoms from, 120
Homeopathy
    overview of, 126–27
    for treating
        allergies, 127
        menopause symptoms, 230
Homocysteine levels, with heart disease,
    146–47, 148
Honey, 58, 69
    Honey-Sweet Broiled Grapefruit Halves,
    259
Hormone replacement therapy (HRT)
    bioidentical, 222–23, 223, 230
    synthetic, 220–22
Horse urine, hormones derived from, 220,
    222
Hostility, cardiovascular health and, 149
Hot flashes, 220, 224
    managing, 225–29, 248
Hover (yoga pose), 99, **99**
HRT. *See* Hormone replacement therapy
Hydrochlorothiazide, for high blood
    pressure, 13
Hypertension, stage 1 and 2, 139. *See also*
    High blood pressure
Hypnosis, for relieving hot flashes, 226
Hypnotherapy, for treating digestive
    problems, 206
Hypoglycemia, nocturnal, 213
Hypothyroidism, 14, 15

I

IBS
    GERD with, 208
    symptoms and diagnosis of, 202–3
    treating, with
        diet, 53, 204–5, 206–7
        supplements, 207

Ice cream
    Strawberry or Peach Coconut Milk Ice
        Cream, 299
IgE antibodies, allergies and, 35, 119, 120
Immune system
    components of, 34
    environmental effects on, 119
    overactive, reasons for, 31
Inactive ingredients, in drugs and
    supplements, 20
Inactivity
    dangers of, 10, 73–75
    prevalence of, 74, 231
Inflammation
    aging process and, 25
    allergies from, 122–23
    causes of, 51, 130, 132
    chronic diseases from, 42, 48
    insulin resistance and, 184, 239
    obesity and, 239
    reducing, with
        antioxidants, 195
        black pepper, 135
        curcumin, 134
        fish oil, 184
        No More Pills Plan, 48
        supplements, 104
        walking, 76
    skin problems from, 187
    stress linked to, 105
Injury, osteoarthritis from, 130
Insomnia
    contributors to, 212, 213, 218–19
        identifying, 214
    drugs to avoid for, 215
    forms of, 212
    treating, with
        aerobic exercise, 216–17
        EFT, 108
        improved sleep hygiene, 217–18
        No More Pills Plan, 214–16
        supplements, 218
        yoga, 217
Insulin resistance
    belly fat increasing, 78
    chronic inflammation and, 184, 239
    in diabetes development, 178
    nuts preventing, 8
Interval training, for blood sugar reduction,
    46, 185, 234
Interval walking, 77–78
Irritable bowel syndrome. *See* IBS

J

Jane iredale mineral foundation, 192

K

Kale
  Hearty Vegetable Soup, 265
  Hearty Winter Harvest Stew, 280
  Roasted Kale Chips, 295
Kidney stones, 65
Kiwifruit, for improving sleep, <u>216</u>
Klonopin, <u>248</u>
Knee pain, treatments for, 19–21, 104, <u>137</u>

L

Label reading, for identifying food allergens,
  <u>20</u>, 43, 253
LAC (acetyl-l-carnitine), for treating
  fibromyalgia, 158
Lactose fillers, in drugs and supplements, <u>20</u>
Lactose intolerance, 37, 55, 56
Laundry soap, for avoiding skin problems,
  192
LDL cholesterol, 141, 148
Leptin, <u>59</u>, 130
Lettuce
  Tangy Roast Beef Lettuce Wraps, 270
Life expectancy, TV watching reducing, 74
Light therapy, for treating
  psoriasis, <u>187</u>
  seasonal affective disorder, <u>175</u>
Liver damage, from statins, 18
Liver problems, coffee preventing, 67
Low-carb diet
  for diabetes prevention or treatment,
    180–81
  No More Pills Plan as, 49
Low-fat diets, drawbacks of, 49, 50, 141–42
Low-glycemic foods, in No More Pills Plan, 51
L-theanine. *See* Theanine
Lunches
  Chicken Noodle Soup with Spinach and
    Basil, 267
  Fish and Chips, 269
  Hearty Vegetable Soup, 265
  Noodle Bowls, 263
  Pan-Seared Fish Tacos, 271
  Roasted Chicken and Spinach Salad, 266
  Salmon Avocado Wraps, 264
  Sweet Potatoes Stuffed with Picadillo, 272
  Tangy Roast Beef Lettuce Wraps, 270
  Warm Sweet Potato and Onion Salad with
    Toasted Walnuts, 268
Lunge, 88–89, **88–89**
Lymphatic system, 34
Lyrica, for fibromyalgia, 154
  side effects of, <u>155</u>

M

Magnesium
  for heart health, 150
  for treating
    diabetes, 183–84
    insomnia, 218
    migraines, 198
Makeup, for concealing skin problems, <u>192</u>
Marrow, in immune system, 34
Massage
  for blood pressure reduction, 140
  for treating headaches and migraines, 197
Meal plan, sample, for No More Pills Plan,
  70–72
Meats. *See also* Beef; Pork
  organic, 50, 58
Medical schools, nutrition education in,
  21–22, 46–47
Meditation
  for blood pressure reduction, 140
  for treating headaches and migraines,
    197–98
Mediterranean diet
  healthy fats in, 50
  for heart health, 142, 145
  for treating
    menopause symptoms, 224
    skin problems, 188
Melatonin, for promoting sleep, 216, 218
Memory loss. *See also* Alzheimer's disease
  case study about, <u>25–26</u>
  from statins, 17
Menopause, preventing osteoporosis during,
  <u>227</u>
Menopause symptoms, 220, 224, 225, <u>228</u>,
  <u>248</u>
  treating, with
    bioidentical hormones, 222–23, <u>223</u>,
      230, <u>248</u>
    homeopathy, 230
    hormone replacement therapy, 220–22
    injectable hormones, <u>228–29</u>
    natural remedies, 225–27
    No More Pills Plan, 223–25
    soy foods, <u>224</u>
    traditional Chinese medicine, 227–29,
      230
Metabolic syndrome, 5, 76
Metformin, for diabetes, <u>12–13</u>, 177, 180
Metta bhavana, for stress reduction, 111,
  112–13
Microbes, in gastrointestinal tract, 205–6
Migraines. *See also* Headaches
  preventing, 195, 197
  treating, 196–200

Tea(s)
  black, health benefits of, 65, 66
  comparisons of, 65–66
  green, health benefits of, 63–65, 66
  herbal, 64
Tension headaches, 193, 200. *See also*
    Headaches
Theanine, for treating
  anxiety, 173
  insomnia, 218
Thought field therapy, 106–7
Thymus, in immune system, 34
Thyroid disease, from fluoridated water, 14,
    15
Tomatoes
  Hearty Vegetable Soup, 265
Traditional Chinese medicine (TCM)
  overview of, 23, 26–28
  for treating
    anxiety and depression, 172
    emotional eating, 240
    headaches and migraines, 196
    menopause symptoms, 227–29, 230
Trans fats, heart disease and, 147–48
Triglycerides, high
  health risks from, 141, 179
  reducing, 62, 145
Triptans, for migraines, 197, 199–200
Tuna
  Tuscan Tuna Cakes, 279
Turkey
  Turkey and Fennel Breakfast Sausage,
    256
Turmeric. *See also* Curcumin
  health benefits of, xi, 61
  for treating arthritis, 134, 136
TV commercials, promoting overeating, 233
TV watching, reducing life expectancy, 74

U

Unilateral Bent-Over Row, 90–91, **90–91**
USDA Organic label, 57
UVB therapy, for treating psoriasis, 187

V

Vegetables. *See also specific vegetables*
  Coconut Vegetable Curry, 278
  fiber in, 49
  for headache prevention, 195
  Hearty Vegetable Soup, 265
  for menopause symptom relief, 225
  organic, 58

Spaghetti Squash with Stir-Fry
    Vegetables, 285
  underconsumption of, 10
  Veggie "Soufflé," 274–75
Vinegar, for lowering blood sugar, 183, 234
Vitamin C
  recommended intake of, 42–43
  for treating allergy symptoms, 125
Vitamin D
  deficiency of, 42, 51, 148–49, 157
  recommended intake of, 42, 51, 150
  for treating
    eczema or psoriasis, 190–91
    fibromyalgia, 157
Vitamin E, for treating allergies, 126
Vitamin K, in parsley, 61
Voluntary image replacement, for treating
    PTSD, 164

W

Walking
  benefits of, 75–76, 79, 97, 235
  for cholesterol reduction, 76, 143
  interval, 77–78, 151
  No More Pills Program for, 78–79, 80–81
  recommended amount of, 77
  water exercise vs., 137
Walking program with interval training, for
    heart health, 151
Wall Pushups, 82
Walnuts
  for cholesterol reduction, 143
  for heart health, 146
  Warm Sweet Potato and Onion Salad with
    Toasted Walnuts, 268
Warrior 2, 100, **100**, 101
Water
  drinking, 62–63
  fluoridation of, 14–15
  in human body, 63
Water exercise program, for knee pain, 104,
    137
Water filters, 15, 29, 63
Weight loss
  exercise for, 234
  from No More Pills Plan, 48, 49, 70,
    233–34
  professional help for, 29
  for relieving hot flashes, 226
Wheat, genetic engineering of, 54
Wild rice, 58
Wine, 58, 69–70, 143
Wraps
  Salmon Avocado Wraps, 264
  Tangy Roast Beef Lettuce Wraps, 270

Y

Yoga
  benefits of, 97
  guidelines for, 97, 101
  poses
    Arm and Leg Extension, 98, **98**
    Cat-Cow, 97, **97**
    Child's Pose, 97, 98, **98**, 101
    Cobra, 99, **99**
    Downward-Facing Dog, 98, **98**, 99, 101
    Hover, 99, **99**
    Plank, 99, **99**
    Reverse Warrior, 100, **100**
    Side Angle, 100, **100**, 101
    Warrior 2, 100, **100**, 101
  for treating insomnia, 217

Z

Zolpidem, avoiding, for insomnia, 19, 215
Zucchini
  Hearty Vegetable Soup, 265